the menopause makeover

The Ultimate Guide to Taking
Control of Your Health and Beauty
During Menopause

STANESS JONEKOS

with WENDY KLEIN, M.D.

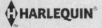

The Menopause Makeover

ISBN-13: 978-0-373-89267-9

Recycling programs for this product may not exist in your area.

Photo credits:
Before Menopause photo by David LaPorte
After Menopause photo by Michael Becker
Staness Jonekos author photo by Michael Becker
Wendy Klein, M.D. author photo by Al Wekelo

www.Harlequin.com

Printed in U.S.A.

The health and medical information provided in this book is not intended to take the place of advice or treatment from your health-care professionals. The authors have worked hard to ensure that the information provided in this book is timely, accurate and helpful. This information should not be considered medical advice. One should consult with her health-care provider. The information provided is for general reference purposes only. Always obtain advice from your physician or other qualified health-care professionals before starting any new treatment.

To my husband, Michael, who showed me
I was lovable before, during and after
menopause.

This book is dedicated to the women before us who
suffered in silence, and to the women stepping out of
the menopause closet today who show the world it's
OK to talk about menopause. Our positive attitude
toward menopause today will pave the path for all
women in the future.

contents

Your Menopause Survival Guide: Eight Steps to a Complete Makeover

| chapter 1 |

Wait a Minute... What Just Happened? Your Body During Menopause

| chapter 2 |

Step One: Okay, So I'm Menopausal... Now What Do I Do? Understanding Your Treatment Options

| chapter 3 |

Step Two: Feeding the New You: How Food Can Set You Free!

| chapter 4 |

**Step Three: Exercise It Off: You Think Hot Flashes
Are Bad? Now It's Time to Burn, Baby, Burn!**   102

| chapter 5 |

**Step Four: Mirror, Mirror on the Wall, Is That Me?
Customizing Your Beauty Routine**   142

| chapter 6 |

**Step Five: Am I Losing My Mind?
Getting Off the Emotional Roller Coaster**   186

PART THREE   333

**Your Menopause Makeover Essential Planner:
12 Weeks to a New You**

Marriage and Menopause?

At forty-seven, I was busy planning my first wedding after thirty years of dating in Los Angeles. It was a joyful time, with the exception of hourly hot flashes, weight gain that made it impossible to preorder the wedding dress of my choice and a vagina that was in no mood for a honeymoon. I was desperate to find solutions to my miserable menopause symptoms so I could feel like myself again, and look like the woman my fiancé fell in love with. I prayed that my doctor would have a magic pill, but she did not.

I began an urgent quest for answers that would allow me to regain control over my health and beauty before the big wedding day. I needed a Menopause Makeover! There were many books and Web sites about menopause, but none had an action plan to guide me through the confusing array of treatment options. During my search, I discovered that the actual process of planning my wedding held the key to my Menopause Makeover. For me, managing menopause was going to take the same amount of effort as planning a wedding.

Since I had less than four months until my wedding, and there were no "menopause makeover" books available, I created a twelve-week plan to manage my uninvited wedding guest—menopause. Inspired by my own wedding planner book, which offered succinct information, checklists, to-do lists, and a place to journal, set goals and track progress, my makeover plan helped me reclaim my health—and my life—in just three months.

I ended up with two planners in my life—one for my wedding and one for my menopause. Marriage and menopause made an odd pair, but the dual-planner approach worked! My menopause makeover plan gave me the direction I needed to accomplish my goals in twelve weeks.

Going through menopause was a wake-up call for me. I could no longer ignore my bad eating habits, lack of exercise, and health issues, such as high blood pressure and fading vision. Most of us are busy with family, career, children, home and parents, with no time left for ourselves. Menopause will demand your attention. Making a commitment to the Twelve-Week Menopause Makeover is the first step to taking control of your health and beauty at midlife. It is the key to a new and revitalized you!

MY STORY: WHY I WROTE THIS BOOK

It took forty-six years for true love to find me and just six months for menopause to seize me. And when I said, "I do" to the man of my dreams, I said, "I don't" to hot flashes, a dry vagina and an ever-expanding waistline.

Menopause hit me at full speed. Before getting married, I decided to get an FSH (follicle-stimulating hormone) test to determine whether or not I was still fertile. I had been on birth control pills for twenty-five years. Getting off the pill to get a "true" FSH test sent my body into chaos. Little did I know that over the years, my "natural" state had started shutting down and had entered a stage of menopause. My FSH test result was 72. Generally, any number over 40 mIU/ML indicates that the ovaries are not producing enough estrogen to keep monthly periods normal (see Chapter 1 for more information).

I was in a state of shock at the results. No one told me how dramatic it would be to experience "the change." When my mother's hormones started changing in her forties, she had a hysterectomy and immediately began taking a hormone therapy drug called Premarin, an oral form of estrogen. My family never saw any "changes" in my mother, other than that she seemed happier. All my friends got married much earlier than I did, had their children, and were nowhere close to menopause. Feeling terribly unprepared, I entered one of the most challenging phases in my life, getting married and "getting" menopause alone.

As any bride knows, the day you get married is the day you want to feel like a princess. We spend months preparing for the big event. Beautifying, pampering, slipping into wedding gowns, hoping to discover the one dress that makes us feel special. I eventually found the perfect gown. But three months before the wedding,

I started gaining weight. I gained seventeen pounds in three months. Just to give you a tiny taste of my dismay, I no longer fit into my wedding gown, and I could not afford to buy another dress two sizes larger.

I was so confused that I started feeling depressed. My fiancé was beyond mystified. What happened to his carefree, loving, supportive, spontaneous and fun wife-to-be? Who was this raging mad woman who "lost it" over the most minor events and attacked him unprovoked? I certainly didn't know. No doubt, the man of my dreams didn't know, either.

Something was wrong. I was not the same person. I was not comfortable in my own skin. All I wanted to do was hide in a cave and hope that when I emerged, the nightmare would be over. I was two sizes bigger, cranky, bloated, sleepless and sweaty. In full panic mode four months before my wedding—the day I had dreamed about my entire life—I scrambled to find answers. It was countdown time, with no room for error. I needed results—and fast! As an executive producer and writer for television, I have a career that requires me to become an expert on many different topics in a short period. Being one of the original executive producers to launch the television network Oxygen Media, cofounded by Oprah Winfrey, I was profoundly committed to producing stories about incredible women, such as Gloria Steinem, Ann Richards, Anna Deavere Smith and Julia-Louis Dreyfus. I had the tools, contacts and passion to find answers.

Desperate, I started reading books, researching the Internet, and speaking to experts. I discovered that nothing was changing but me! I was doing everything the menopause books and Internet articles suggested, from dieting to exercising, yet nothing seemed to be working. I searched online and in bookstores for the one book that would explain what was happening to me and show me the way out. I read nearly fifty books, but even though they were loaded with all the medical information I needed to understand menopause, none gave me the solution—the program—that I needed to take back my life. What was a menopausal bride to do? I wanted one-stop shopping. I wanted an ultimate plan. And it was up to me to create it.

Inspired by the wedding planner books I used for my wedding, I decided I really needed a menopause planner to help me keep track of hormones, exercise and my diet the same way I kept track of caterers, florists and dress fittings. Through extensive research, interviews with medical experts and trial and error, I developed an eight-step program and menopause planner that really worked. My menopause planner gave me the tools I needed to look and feel better in twelve short weeks, and it will do the same for you.

This book is your survival guide to menopause. It will take the mystery out of menopause, offer you proven solutions to your symptoms, and help you stay sane and organized. With my twelve-week program for managing symptoms and regaining your health and beauty, you will feel like yourself again in no time!

Thanks to this unusual combination of life transitions—marriage and menopause—I discovered a wonderful connection: Just as you commit to loving the partner of your dreams, you need to commit to loving yourself. This is especially true during menopause. With The Menopause Makeover, you can say "I do" to the new you.

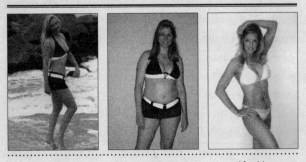

Before Menopause   During Menopause   After My Menopause Makeover

MY COMMITMENT TO YOU

The Menopause Makeover produced incredible results, and everyone wanted to know my secret. After my wedding day, I repeated the 12-Week Plan with great success. Knowing that I couldn't be the only one having trouble with menopause, I decided to share what I'd learned to help other women manage menopause. Taking this commitment seriously, I launched a Web site and Hot Flash newsletter to reach out to menopausal women worldwide. The first month, over ten thousand women searching for menopause solutions found the Web site, women from the U.S.A., Great Britain, Canada, the Bahamas, and Australia. They openly shared their frustrations and concerns. Women wrote to my advice column, "Dear Crabby," revealing their deepest fears. I discovered that women were struggling most with weight gain and aging, the very same frustrations I was experiencing. Miserable menopause symptoms, like hot flashes and dry skin, usually came second or third on the list of menopause complaints.

Hearing from other women going through menopause helped me refine the Menopause Makeover program to encompass all their needs and concerns. The Menopause Makeover offers eating and exercise advice, beauty tips, and emotional and relationship support, topped off with a splash of spirituality and a dash of happiness—you need to work on all areas of your life in order to truly manage menopause.

Before publishing this book I spent two years fine-tuning the program, collaborating with medical experts and eventually teaming up with a leading expert on menopause, Dr. Wendy Klein, Associate Professor of Medicine, Obstetrics & Gynecology at Virginia Commonwealth University School of Medicine. As a pioneer in women's health, Dr. Klein shared my passion for helping women manage menopause. We spent months discussing menopause symptoms and treatment solutions, from complementary remedies to hormone therapy, along with the latest scientific evidence on hormone therapy, bioidenticals and compounded hormones. We read the latest studies from the Women's

Health Initiative and leading medical journals on risks associated with hormone therapy, from heart disease to cancer. I was astonished at the misinformation out there in bookstores and online!

Dr. Klein's dedication to accuracy ensures that you have the most up-to-date information at your fingertips. In order to design your own successful Menopause Makeover, you need to be informed and understand all your choices. In her mission to educate both practitioners and patients, Dr. Klein is committed to healthy solutions based on sound scientific research. I discovered that traditional medicine is not only aggressively researching treatment choices for women, but there are already many FDA-approved options available, all of which are discussed in this book.

There's a lot of confusion out there about menopause treatment—what's safe, what isn't, what works and what doesn't. With the help of Dr. Klein, this book provides clear, simple explanations about menopause symptoms and treatment choices. The Menopause Makeover is more than a girlfriend's guide to menopause; it is a book built on a foundation of sound science. This book is dedicated to your menopausal journey. You have all the tools needed in The Menopause Makeover to go through "the change" informed with the latest scientific evidence, so you can celebrate your new beginning.

THE MENOPAUSE MAKEOVER IS FOR YOU

When the word *menopause* is used in this book, I am speaking to all women going through perimenopause, menopause, postmenopause and surgical menopause. If you picked up this book, you are probably suffering from uncomfortable menopausal symptoms and you are looking for:

- Easy-to-understand explanations about what is happening to your ever-changing body and mind
- Treatment options
- New ways of eating and exercising
- Beauty tips that will make you look and feel better
- Solutions to your cranky moods
- Tips that can make sex more enjoyable
- Motivation to accomplish your goals
- A customized plan for surviving—and thriving through—menopause
- Control over your health, your beauty, and your life

Menopause is a natural transition in a woman's life. Yet, it may be the one event that we are least prepared for. From puberty to marriage to new careers to children, each transition is celebrated. We responsibly go through our adult lives taking care of others—our partners, children, family, friends, bosses, coworkers and community—with little time left for ourselves. It is understandable that when you reach menopause, it can be overwhelming and confusing. After all, menopause is frustrating! All of a sudden you're dealing with unappealing body changes, uncontrollable crankiness, impatience toward the ones you love, thinning hair, an ever-expanding waistline, difficulty concentrating and those uninvited hot flashes.

The good news is that it is time to take care of you. Menopause is a time for personal growth, lifestyle changes and new solutions. Unfortunately, nobody gave us a map to navigate this journey in life. You may feel completely out of control, but you can create balance and find joy in the new vibrant you. This book will offer you individual options—from hormone choices to eating and exercise plans. Because we all experience menopause differently, you must create a plan that fits your needs.

You are not alone. By the year 2020, the number of U.S. women older than 51 (the average age menopause can occur naturally), is expected to be more than 50 million. According to the North American Menopause Society, every day an estimated six thousand women have reached menopause in North America—that's over 2 million a year! Currently, almost 20 percent of female baby boomers are slamming into one of the stages of menopause. Approximately 75 percent of these women will experience uncomfortable symptoms, such as hot flashes, weight gain, fuzzy thinking and low sex drive, which can lead to irritability. You are not losing your mind. Rather, you are gaining an opportunity to create new beginnings!

Whether your menopause symptoms are mild or severe, this planner will help you feel better and take charge of your health. Menopause is more than fluctuating hormones and hot flashes; it is a time to look at all aspects of your life. It is the beginning of a new chapter and an opportunity for self-renewal. Are you happy? Is it time for a tune-up? Or a major overhaul? It was for me.

I made a number of startling discoveries during my 12-Week Menopause Makeover—some exciting, some discouraging. It became clear that I needed to exercise five to six days a week to be healthy. I had to eat more protein and fewer pastries, and cut my portions. My skin-care routine had to be modified. My unhealthy relationships had to be addressed. I had to create a partnership with my doctor. And my self-image had to be readjusted. I had to get comfortable in my new skin.

Transitions can be scary and exciting; it is how we look at the journey that makes the difference. Planning a wedding can be stressful, yet it is also joyful, a time of celebration. Why can't the menopausal transition—complete with its undesirable symptoms and midlife changes—be an exciting time, a time of celebration, too? A new beginning? If we throw parties for Sweet Sixteen, graduation, bridal showers and baby showers, we should throw hot-flash parties as well!

HOW TO USE THIS BOOK

When you are planning a wedding, there is a clear-cut agenda and time line, a team to help you, and a list of choices to make and questions to answer. No two weddings are alike; it's up to you to design the wedding of your dreams. This book utilizes a similar step-by-step strategy, incorporating tips, checklists and calendars to help you design a personal action plan—a Menopause Makeover designed by you, for you.

THE THREE-PART PROGRAM

The Menopause Makeover is an easy-to-use three-part process.

PART ONE, "Your Menopause Survival Guide" is the powerful 8-step program. These eight steps are the actual makeover—your physical, emotional and spiritual program to look and feel better. Each chapter in Part One will give you the information you need to be successful, complete with helpful charts and checklists.

PART TWO, "Your Menopause Makeover: Planning your Transformation" gives you the tools to customize your makeover. In Part Two, you'll take stock of where you are today and set personal goals for your 12-week makeover.

PART THREE, "Your Menopause Makeover Essential Planner: Twelve Weeks to a New You" provides you with all the tools you need to achieve your makeover goals. Part Three is your essential planner. It includes the forms you need to keep on track, self-assessments to chart your progress, and delicious recipes to feed the new you. Documenting your journey can be rewarding, especially when you start to see the results.

After I said, "I do" to this Menopause Makeover plan, I never looked back. When I started on this journey, I had a long way to go. I had to learn to love the new me. I had to learn to be grateful for what I had.

I had to learn to be compassionate toward myself, yet determined to make changes. I had to admit that I was starting to age (gulp), and that was a biggie. Today, I feel more vibrant and sexier than ever before. It took hard work, but with this 12-Week, 8-step program I was able to see the areas where I was failing, and the areas that were working well.

If you're struggling through menopause as I was, and want to feel better, look better and be healthy, then The Menopause Makeover is for you. If you do the work, you will see the results. Trust me—if I could do it, you can, too!

QUIZ Are you ready for a Menopause Makeover?	YES	NO
1 > Have you gained more than ten pounds in the past year?	☐	☐
2 > Have you tried other diets without success?	☐	☐
3 > Are you perimenopausal, menopausal or newly postmenopausal?	☐	☐
4 > Are you experiencing menopausal symptoms, such as hot flashes?	☐	☐
5 > Have you lost your waistline?	☐	☐
6 > Do you make excuses for not wanting to have sex?	☐	☐
7 > Do you have cravings for sugar, salt, or alcohol?	☐	☐

QUIZ	Are you ready for a Menopause Makeover?	YES	NO
8 >	Are you hungry all the time?		
9 >	Are you not seeing results like you used to from exercise?		
10 >	Are you depressed?		
11 >	Are you buying bigger clothes this year?		
12 >	Are you between the ages forty and sixty?		
13 >	Do you feel like the "normal" you is a thing of the past?		
14 >	Are you cranky and irritable?		
15 >	Do you have less patience for loved ones?		

If you answered "**YES**" to at least 10 of the above
questions, it is time to regain
control of your health and beauty again. It is time to
start *The Menopause Makeover!*

PART ONE

Your Menopause Survival Guide:
Eight Steps to a
Complete Makeover

chapter 1

Wait a Minute... What Just Happened? Your Body During Menopause

Feeling blue, gaining weight, suffering from hot flashes, being cranky, losing interest in sex and forgetting things—this had become my new daily reality. And as if that were not enough, I had to start slathering on gallons of facial moisturizer, hoping my once-radiant complexion would return.

Feeling helpless, frustrated and desperate for a solution, I scheduled an appointment to see my doctor. After the examination and a tearful discussion, including my confession—"I think I am losing my mind"—the doctor gave me an FSH blood test. Praying I didn't have a strange disease causing all this misery, I eagerly awaited the results.

A week later, the doctor phoned and said, "I have good news. You're not losing your mind. You don't have a disease. You're going through menopause."

I said, "What! I'm *what?* Not me? Wait a minute... what just happened?"

Shocked, standing there with the phone in my hand, I felt as if life as I knew it was over. Menopause had never even occurred to me; I was totally blindsided. Surely this was not happening to *me*. My favorite blouse was suddenly drenched from an uninvited hot flash. My mind was fuzzy as I tried to focus on the clock pounding over the kitchen sink—*tick, tock, tick, tock*—or was that my heart? It certainly wasn't my egg count—that was now *tocked!*

I was scared—something I took for granted had just been taken away without my permission. The sunlight was streaming through the kitchen window, giving me a glimmer of hope that there must be a way to make this go away. I took a deep breath, and said, "Okay, give me something to fix this."

Well, the hard truth is that there is no magic pill that will "fix" menopause. Believe me, I tried to find one. The good news is that you can manage menopause. The first step is to understand your symptoms and your treatment options. If you know your options, you can manage menopause.

You may be feeling miserable and frustrated, wanting to feel "normal" again—and fast. Fortunately, you have a big advantage in your life that you may not be acknowledging—unlike other transitions, now you have a lifetime of experience at hand! You are already equipped with survival tools and coping skills. You managed to make it through puberty, perhaps marriage, divorce, children, financial challenges, family issues, and career ups and downs. If you have gotten this far in life, hot flashes, a few new wrinkles, a declining libido and weight gain are all conditions you can handle. You are armed with a lifetime of knowledge. Once you make up your mind to meet these issues head-on, you are ready to walk through a new door and realize your new powerful potential!

WHAT IS MENOPAUSE?

As I urgently searched for answers to my severe menopause symptoms and cranky moods, it occurred to me that this was a time in my life that demanded attention. The word *menopause* took on a new meaning for me: ME-NO-PAUSE. I could no longer give all my attention to others. I now had to focus on "ME." I could "NO" longer "PAUSE" on matters regarding "ME."

Menopause is actually derived from the Greek roots *meno* (month) and *pausis* (a pause, a cessation). Menopause, the natural stopping of your reproductive cycle, is a completely normal physical transition in a woman's life. The dictionary defines *menopause* as "the time in a woman's life when menstruation diminishes and ceases, usually between the ages of 45 and 55."

The menopause journey has three stages. Perimenopause (*peri* is Latin meaning "around" or "near") is the time prior to the cessation of menstruation, when you begin to experience hormonal changes and you are still having intermittent periods. Many doctors now refer to perimenopause as the menopausal transition. I will refer to it this way as well. You have reached menopause once you have gone 12 months without a period. Postmenopause is the time after menopause when the acute symptoms of estrogen absence generally diminish.

Going through the menopausal transition is the reverse of puberty. Puberty was the transition in your life when your hormones were gearing up for the reproductive years. Remember your first period? Emotional outbursts, tender breasts, restless nights and feeling bloated?

THREE STAGES OF MENOPAUSE

Perimenopause: The phase leading up to menopause when your hormones start changing. In this stage, you may experience symptoms such as hot flashes and irregular periods. This transition can last up to six years.

Menopause: Once you have gone 12 months without a period, you are considered to be in menopause.

Postmenopause: The years after you've reached menopause.

YOUR HORMONES DURING MENOPAUSE

During the transition into menopause, you may experience many of the same puberty symptoms, but for different reasons. Instead of turning on your hormones, your body is now turning them off by slowly producing less estrogen and progesterone.

THE LEADING LADY AND COSTARS OF MENOPAUSE

Estrogen is the feminizing hormone responsible for maintaining the health of the reproductive tissue, the breasts, the skin and the brain. Estrogen is secreted mostly from the ovaries. We make three types of estrogen:

Estradiol: The dominant, most biologically active estrogen produced by the ovaries before menopause.

Estrone: The most abundant estrogen made by your body after menopause—less potent than estradiol. Before menopause it was produced by your ovaries but was inactive.

Estriol: Increases during pregnancy—less potent than estradiol.

Progesterone is a hormone produced by the ovaries and by the placenta. Progesterone helps prepare the uterus for pregnancy. When you are pregnant, progesterone also stimulates the mammary glands and maintains the pregnancy.

Testosterone, another hormone secreted by the ovaries and the adrenal glands, started slowing down before menopause. It influences your energy and libido. Men generate over 20 times more testosterone than women. The ovaries and adrenal glands produce testosterone. After menopause we produce about half the amount of testosterone.

Follicle-stimulating hormone (FSH) is secreted by the pituitary gland, and triggers the growth of eggs in the ovaries and estrogen production starting the ovulation cycle.

Luteinizing hormone (LH) is secreted by the pituitary gland and stimulates ovulation.

Many women who had severe symptoms during puberty may also have a challenging menopause, while women who slid through adolescence easily often have the same experience with menopause. We are all different, and menopause is no exception. In order to fully understand menopause, we must look at how our bodies have been operating since birth.

We are born with a finite number of eggs, about 1 to 2 million, stored in small follicles in our ovaries. From birth to puberty, the majority of eggs will die. At puberty, about 400,000 remain. Each month in which we have a period, about 1,000 eggs are lost and usually only 1 actually matures into a fertile egg (ovum). A woman will have about 500 ovulations.

The ovaries not only hold these eggs, but also produce the hormones estrogen and progesterone. During days 1 to 14 of your cycle, a hormone called follicle-stimulating hormone (FSH) is produced by the pituitary gland in your brain. It stimulates the growth of immature follicles to maturation and it stimulates the production of estrogen. Once there is a sufficient level of estrogen in your body, usually around day 12 to 16 of your cycle, the pituitary gland sends luteinizing hormone (LH) to signal the follicle to release the egg (ovulation).

Once ovulation has occurred, your estrogen levels drop and progesterone starts to rise. By day 20, progesterone levels are high enough to prepare the uterus for pregnancy. If the egg is fertilized, your progesterone levels will remain high. If the egg is not fertilized, both estrogen and progesterone levels fall and you start your period. This process is called the menstrual cycle. During menopause, your body begins to produce less estrogen and progesterone, causing this cycle to become irregular, and eventually ending.

WHY DOES MENOPAUSE OCCUR?

Since you're born with a finite number of eggs, the number of follicles in your ovaries decreases over time. The ovaries also start to produce lower levels of hormones. Menopause occurs when the ovaries stop making enough hormones to stimulate your monthly cycle.

SO HOW DO I KNOW IT'S MENOPAUSE?

As your hormones start changing and your body enters the menopausal transition, there are a number of factors that will help confirm whether you are experiencing symptoms associated with perimenopause or menopause. If you think you are experiencing one of the stages of menopause, visit your doctor or healthcare practitioner. This is a perfect time to reassess your health and to be proactive about preventive measures and health screening.

Communicating with your clinician is important. You need to give her all the information she needs to make an accurate evaluation. Next, you will review different treatment options. It will take a joint effort with your practitioner to successfully diagnose and manage your menopause. If your symptoms are not being properly treated, seek a second opinion. The North American Menopause Society has a resource that lists knowledgeable doctors belonging to the organization. (See the Author's Note at the back of this book.)

MAKING THE MOST OF YOUR DOCTOR'S VISIT

Be prepared! Here are helpful tips on how to provide your practitioner with the information she needs to make an accurate diagnosis and evaluate your symptoms, making the most out of your visit.

{ Before your appointment: }

- List your current symptoms and their severity level.

- Note your menstrual patterns.

- List all recent medical issues and physical concerns.

- List your personal medical history.

- List your family medical history.

- Make a list of *all* medications, vitamins and supplements you are currently taking.

- Think about treatment choices ahead of time and come prepared with questions to ask.

{ After your physical examination: }

- Ask if your personal or family medical history will influence your treatment choices.

- Discuss having a follicle-stimulating hormone (FSH) blood test.

- Discuss other medical testing you may need at this stage of your life, such as mammograms, bone density testing, colonoscopy and lipid profiles.

After you discuss your medical history, testing, treatment options and current medications, and you decide on a course of action, make sure to ask your doctor about side effects, benefits, risks and length of treatment. Also discuss your risk of postmenopausal osteoporosis and whether you still need to practice birth control.

For helpful forms to prepare for your appointment, see Chapter 13, "The Essential Planner."

In order to make the most of your doctor's visit, it's helpful to come prepared.

Bring the list of suggested information from "Making the Most of Your Doctor's Visit" to your next appointment. This information will help facilitate your conversation and result in a more thorough evaluation. Menopause can be a complex transition. The more information your practitioner has the better the odds of properly managing your menopause symptoms.

It is important for you to trust your health practitioner and feel comfortable discussing anything from sex to hot flashes. A good relationship will be rewarding in the long run.

MENOPAUSE TESTS

Your practitioner may decide to give you a blood test to determine where you are in the menopause process. There are a number of different tests available. The most reliable test is the follicle-stimulating hormone blood test.

FSH (Follicle-Stimulating Hormone) Blood Level Test

The FSH (follicle-stimulating hormone) blood level test is a simple blood sample that can be taken at your doctor's office or at a lab. As the number of follicles decline over the years, your FSH levels rise. If you still get your period, you should have this test on the third to fifth day of your period. If you no longer get a period, you can take this test at any time. Since hormone levels fluctuate, it is often a good idea to repeat this blood test in one to three months to confirm the results.

The FSH blood test is generally a good indicator as to where you are in the menopause transition. A higher number indicates that you are closer to menopause. When your FSH is elevated, it is a sign that your pituitary is working hard to stimulate ovulation, even when the ovaries are no longer able to ovulate in response.

WHAT DO THE RESULTS MEAN?

Perimenopause: Levels above 25 mIU/ml (milli-international units per milliliter) likely signal that the ovaries are just starting to cease estrogen production.

Menopause: FSH levels of 40 or above generally indicate that your ovaries aren't producing enough estrogen to maintain your monthly cycle. You may still get your periods intermittently even though your ovaries have started to decrease their hormonal activity.

Postmenopause: Levels 40 to 135.

There is some variability among laboratories—
your clinician will be able to interpret the results.

HORMONE BLOOD LEVEL TESTS

Many doctors test individual hormones, such as estradiol or testosterone. Hormones vary significantly from day to day, and from individual to individual, so these are not generally useful tests when treating menopause symptoms, as your hormone levels often won't correspond to symptoms.

URINE AND SALIVA HOME TESTS

There are also urine and saliva tests you can do at home to check your FSH and hormone levels. Although popular, these tests are not as accurate as the FSH blood test, and there is no sound scientific evidence to guide their use.

Because your body and hormones are changing daily, a simple FSH blood test may be a useful step to a correct diagnosis. That being said, no one test can accurately evaluate your menopause status. Your body is constantly changing, and your symptoms may change. To properly "test" for menopause, your practitioner should review your overall health profile.

UNDERSTANDING YOUR MENOPAUSE SYMPTOMS

Once you establish that you are in one of the stages of menopause, understanding your symptoms is the first step to managing them. Your symptoms can give you clues as to what your body is experiencing. This will help when deciding what course of action to pursue. Some women will experience very troubling symptoms, while others slide through the menopause transition without a hot flash. How you experience and manage your transition will be unique to you. We are all different!

Tracking your symptoms may be the most useful information used in treating menopause. Your body is giving you clues that you can use to restore balance. Just as a detective collects evidence to solve a case, you, too, can collect information and solve *your* case.

Your symptoms will guide you throughout your menopausal journey as they continue to change until postmenopause. We all know that experiencing menopause symptoms can be challenging, but it can be fascinating to witness your body's sophisticated orchestration between you and your hormones.

Compare the complex mechanisms in a watch to the effects hormones have on our body. A watch has many interlocking gears. One turns the other. Some are big and some are small. When one does not function properly, it causes a cascading effect on the others. Similarly, the interplay of reproductive hormones is extremely complex; they affect one another. Often your symptoms will tell you what "gear" is out of whack, so you can adopt the best approach.

Document your symptoms using this checklist before starting your Menopause Makeover. Revisit this checklist in three months after completing the 12-Week Plan. Are your symptoms better? Worse? Do you have new symptoms? Many symptoms experienced during the menopausal transition are hormone-related, but many are age-related. Once you document your current menopause symptom status, use this information to discuss treatment options with your health-care provider. If your symptoms are mild and tolerable, they are likely to be resolved without any treatment at all.

SYMPTOMS CHECKLIST

Do you experience any of these symptoms? If so, check off the symptoms that apply to you and rate the level of intensity, with 1 being mild and 10 being miserable, then record the date. Use this checklist to discuss your symptoms with your doctor.

PHYSICAL SIGNS	Intensity (1-10)	Date
Irregular periods		
Hot flashes		
Night sweats		
Weight gain		
Breast tenderness		
Heart palpitations		
Migraine headaches		
Bladder changes		
Incontinence		
Vaginal dryness		
Joint aches		
Muscle tension		
Skin changes		
Hair changes		
Fluid retention & bloating		

PSYCHOLOGICAL SIGNS	Intensity (1-10)	Date
Mood swings		
Crankiness		
Memory loss		
Sleep problems		
Loss of libido		
Depression		
Fatigue		
Anxiety		

What menopausal symptoms are you experiencing?
Many of the symptoms you're experiencing are very common for menopausal women. You're not alone! The following lists the causes and solutions for the most common symptoms—go through it and note which symptoms you've been experiencing. Speak to your practitioner about the approach that might be right for you.

IRREGULAR PERIODS
This is probably the first symptom you noticed. When you begin to go through menopause, your periods start to get a bit unpredictable. You may notice spotting, heavier or lighter bleeding and your periods may be longer or shorter.

CAUSES: When the ovaries run out of functioning eggs and hormone secretion is erratic, your natural cycle changes. Some months you may ovulate and some months you may not.

SOLUTIONS: Keep track of your periods in the Essential Planner. What date does your period start? How long does it last? Is bleeding heavy or light? Are you suffering from cramps? When appropriate, a low dose of birth control pills can regulate your periods, with the added benefit of birth control.

HOT FLASHES

The most common and the most irritating symptom associated with menopause is hot flashes. As many as 75 percent of women going through menopause experience hot flashes. A hot flash is a feeling of warmth to intense heat on the upper body and face lasting 1 to 5 minutes, sometimes followed by chills. Your heart rate can also increase, up to 7 to 15 beats more per minute.

CAUSES: Those ever-changing hormones cause hot flashes. When estrogen levels fall, your body's thermostat, located in the brain (hypothalamus), may have a hard time regulating your body temperature. Some women are more sensitive than others to this temperature change. We are all different, so frequency, duration and intensity may vary. The good news is that hot flashes usually decline two years after postmenopause, although some women have them longer.

There are also nonhormonal causes for hot flashes. Being overweight, smoking, suffering from diabetes,

infection, malignancies, autoimmune disorders, under-
or overactive thyroid and some medications, such as
SERMs or SSRIs, can also cause hot flashes. Yet, even
the healthiest person, living a stress-free lifestyle, can
experience hot flashes. There is nothing fun about hot
flashes. They usually come on at the most inconvenient
times.

SOLUTIONS: There is hope! Start documenting the times
you suffer from hot flashes in your daily planner. Are
they triggered by alcohol? Spicy foods? Caffeine? Heat?
Smoking cigarettes? Are you asleep? Are you under
stress? Determine your hot flash triggers and avoid
them. Wear layered clothing. Sip a cool beverage. Sit
near the air conditioner. Carry a cute hand fan. Being
prepared is your first course of action. Often low-dose
hormone therapy (HT) can bring hot-flash relief. Other
medications, including antidepressants, antiseizure
drugs and some herbs may also be helpful in relieving
hot flashes. Enjoy a yoga class, schedule a massage or
a relaxing bath. Regular exercise is a must, and you
should maintain a healthy weight. If you smoke, stop!
Review your medications with your clinician and make
sure they are not causing or aggravating hot flashes.

NIGHT SWEATS

When you're sleeping, it is normal for your body temperature to drop slightly. However, thrashing around in
bed all night from uncomfortable nighttime sweating,
followed by a cold sensation, can be a drag and promise
a day of irritability.

CAUSES: Low or fluctuating hormone levels can disturb the body's thermostat for many.

If you wake up sweating, that cooling system in your brain is stimulating the sweat glands.

SOLUTIONS: Sleep in cotton PJs on cotton sheets. Set up an electric fan next to your side of the bed, and lower your thermostat before going to bed. Avoid caffeine drinks, and consume no alcohol or nicotine close to bedtime. Sleep at regular hours. Make sure your bedroom is dark, and keep the temperature cool. Exercise daily, but not within three hours of bedtime. If you are experiencing stress, meditate and relax.

WEIGHT GAIN

One of the most frustrating symptoms during menopause is weight gain. The average woman gains one pound per year starting around the age of 40, for a total of about five to ten additional pounds, thanks to aging and a lower metabolism.

CAUSES: Only some weight gain can be blamed on our changing hormones. Over the years, many of us have had less time to exercise and eat properly, and when we enter menopause the effects are unforgiving. During menopause, it is natural for the body to store fat around your "middle," so that your waistline starts to disappear. It is often typical to gain 5 to 10 pounds during the menopause transition, but more than that suggests the need to make changes in your lifestyle!

SOLUTIONS: A commitment to healthy food choices and daily exercise is a vital step toward feeling better and taking control of your health. *Menopausal weight gain is a wake-up call.* Set weight goals and track your weight for the next 12 weeks in the Essential Planner. More information and solutions to weight gain are found in Chapter 3.

BREAST TENDERNESS

Breast tissue is sensitive to hormonal change and can sometimes feel tender. Many women notice tender breasts when they first begin hormone therapy.

CAUSES: Hormonal changes may cause fluid retention in your breasts, similar to your monthly cycle experience. Once your hormones are stabilized, you will notice this uncomfortable symptom subsiding.

SOLUTIONS: Cut back on your caffeine and salt consumption.

HEART PALPITATIONS

Have you ever felt as if your heart were pounding out of your chest? During menopause, heart palpitations can be scary and can happen at inappropriate times. Sometimes palpitations accompany hot flashes. This double whammy is no fun.

CAUSES: No one knows for sure why some women suffer from heart palpitations during menopause. It is often attributed to hormonal fluctuation.

SOLUTIONS: If you suspect heart disease or if heart disease runs in your family, be sure to discuss these symptoms with your health-care provider.

MIGRAINE HEADACHES

If migraine headaches are new to you, or if they only happened during the first few days of your period or during ovulation, you may be responding to changing estrogen levels. Do you have triggers? Alcohol? Temperature change? Stress? Dieting? Caffeine? Certain foods? Medications? Are you suffering from a sinus infection, have dental issues or allergies? Migraines that appear during menopause will often subside during postmenopause.

CAUSES: Some studies have established a connection between migraines and menstrual periods for some women. During perimenopause, fluctuating estrogen levels may trigger more migraines than you experienced during a normal cycle.

SOLUTIONS: Leveling hormones alleviates migraines for some women; but for others, hormone therapy makes the headaches worse. If you have tension headaches, nonprescription medications, such as aspirin, or anti-inflammatory medications (such as ibuprofen) can offer relief. Do you have triggers? Alcohol? Spicy foods? Stress? Practice stress management and relaxation techniques. Small studies have suggested that riboflavin, magnesium and/or coenzyme Q_{10} are supplements that may help reduce your migraines, if taken daily. Prescription medicines are available to help with migraines. Speak to your clinician about your options.

BLADDER CHANGES/INCONTINENCE

There is nothing worse than panicking to find a bath-room when you've gotta go. Up to 60 percent of all women 45 to 55 years of age suffer from mild incontinence, so you are not alone.

CAUSES: Common culprits are age, obesity, family history, childbearing trauma, hysterectomy and smoking/chronic coughing.

SOLUTIONS: Before visiting your health-care provider, keep a 3-day diary, recording how many times a day you urinate, whether the urge wakes you up at night, whether urine leaks out before you get to the bathroom or when you sneeze or cough. Also record your fluid intake. Wear a light minipad; it is much easier to change than your panties or slacks. Make sure you pee after every meal. Treatments for incontinence include Kegel exercises, avoiding bladder irritants (caffeine, soda, tomatoes, grapefruit juice), fluid restriction, bladder training and urination at timed intervals.

VAGINAL DRYNESS

Vaginal dryness is not only a common menopause symptom, it can actually affect your sexual desire and pleasure. With dryness, your vagina can become irritated more easily from friction, and the vaginal tissues may lose their elasticity.

CAUSES: When your estrogen levels drop, vaginal dryness can occur. Estrogen plumps up the cells in the vaginal wall so they produce more lubrication.

SOLUTIONS: For a quick fix, try a bioadhesive lubricant, such as Astroglide or a vaginal moisturizer, such as Replens. Estrogen improves lubrication, keeping vaginal tissues working properly. Low-dose hormone therapy or estrogen creams applied vaginally may alleviate vaginal dryness. If you suffer from a number of menopause symptoms, oral hormone therapy may be a better option. For more information, see Chapter 7.

SKIN CHANGES

No one escapes the aging process. Sun damage, smoking, eating poorly and inadequate skin care are big contributors to sagging and wrinkling skin. If you loved getting a summer suntan, the effects of sun on your skin are damaging. Gravity takes its toll on everyone who has spent 40-plus years on this planet, but what most of us notice during menopause is that the elasticity and firmness of our skin decreases.

CAUSES: The skin is supported by collagen and elastin fibers, which are supported by estrogen. Hormone changes can affect the skin's physiology, with almost 30 percent of the skin's collagen depleted over the first five years after menopause.

SOLUTIONS: Wear sunscreen with a sun protection factor (SPF) of 15+ daily—this is not negotiable if you want healthy skin. Antioxidants and topical retinoids can help sun-damaged skin. Exfoliate regularly and moisturize daily. This is a perfect time for a new skin regimen. For more skin-care information, including nonsurgical cosmetic treatments, see Chapter 5.

HAIR CHANGES

During menopause, 40 to 50 percent of women report some hair loss or thinning, called androgenic alopecia (AGA). Perhaps, you're sprouting facial hair. Is it coarse? Does it appear on your chin, upper lip and cheeks? Then you may be one of the 5 to 15 percent of women who experience hirsutism (presence of excess hair). Some women experience excessive peach fuzz or discover rogue hairs.

CAUSES: Having too much or too little hair during midlife can be caused by changing hormones, age, genetics, metabolism, high blood pressure medication, depression, thyroid disease, chemotherapy or stress. Androgenic alopecia (AGA) or hair thinning is often genetic. Did your mom or dad have thinning hair?

SOLUTIONS: To treat hair thinning, try topical minoxidil solution (Rogaine 2%). It is the only over-the-counter drug available to promote hair growth in women with androgenic alopecia.

If you only have a few rogue hairs, try tweezing, shaving, depilatory hair creams or waxing. Dark peach fuzz can often be treated with facial bleach products or waxing. Electrolysis is another option. Vaniqa cream (not available in Canada) is a prescription topical enzyme inhibitor of hair growth. For more information, see Chapter 5.

FLUID RETENTION AND BLOATING

Remember feeling bloated during your period? As if a few days a month weren't bad enough, when you go through the menopausal transition, this can persist for months on end!

CAUSES: The causes of bloating vary. Irregular ovarian function and fluctuating estrogen levels during menopause can cause bloating. Poor nutrition and high salt intake can also cause bloating.

SOLUTIONS: In the Essential Planner, note the days you feel bloated and decrease your salt intake those days. A high-potassium diet may help provide for bloating relief. High-potassium foods include all meats, poultry and fish, apricots, avocado, banana, cantaloupe, kiwi, lima beans, milk, oranges, potatoes, prunes, spinach, tomatoes and winter squash.

MOOD SWINGS AND CRANKINESS

Are you experiencing a lot of change and stress lately? Midlife stressors, such as relationship issues, losses, caring for parents or career issues, can all make you moody.

CAUSES: Hormonal flux can make the best of us moody and cranky. Throw in hot flashes, weight gain and a dry vagina—no wonder you're moody and cranky!

SOLUTIONS: If you are experiencing mood swings, this is a good time in your life to start making time to relax, meditate, practice yoga, enjoy herbal teas and pamper yourself. Exercise and good nutrition will help. For more information, see Chapter 6.

MEMORY LOSS

Forget your car keys? Forget an appointment? Repeat the same thing a few times only to be corrected by your listener? Short-term memory loss or fuzzy thinking is common during menopause.

CAUSES: The effects of estrogen, age, stress, medications and a decline in overall health may all affect your memory. Fluctuating hormones can alter the connections in your brain, short-circuiting your memory. Night sweats, lack of sleep, midlife stress and hot flashes can all contribute to memory loss.

SOLUTIONS: Ask your loved ones for support. Get organized with planners, calendars and PDAs. Keep your mind active, and enjoy a healthy lifestyle. Make sure you get a good night's sleep. A rested mind can absorb more information. To find out more, see Chapter 6.

SLEEP PROBLEMS

If you are experiencing night sweats, it is no surprise that you are not sleeping at night. A sleepless night will promise a day of irritability and mood swings. Nonmenopausal sleep problems can also contribute to sleepless nights. Consuming food, caffeine or alcohol just before bedtime, and bad habits like watching TV in bed can also keep you awake.

CAUSES: Anxiety, mood swings, hot flashes, itchy skin and suffering from depression can all contribute to sleepless nights.

SOLUTIONS: Avoid stimulants, such as exercise and caffeine in the evening, and no excessive daytime napping.

If your sleepless nights are caused by menopause symptoms, a low-dose hormone therapy may bring back restful sleep. Prescription sleep aids are another option. Discuss those with your health-care provider. Keep a "sleep diary" in your 12-Week Planner under "Notes." Track the time you fell asleep, the time you woke up, what you ate before sleeping and how many times you woke up during the night.

LOSS OF LIBIDO

Not feeling sexy? Between the ages of 55 and 65, sexual desire may diminish for both men and women. Once we exit the reproducing stage of our life, we may experience a loss of libido.

CAUSES: Aging, along with changing hormone levels, may blow the flame of desire out of your love life. Declining levels of estrogen and testosterone may also contribute to decreased libido. Suffering from menopause symptoms, including vaginal dryness, may quash any interest in sex. Refer to "vaginal dryness" in Chapter 7. Physical, emotional and social factors can all affect your libido. Certain medications for blood pressure, depression, heart disease or diabetes can decrease your libido as well.

SOLUTIONS: Discuss your declining libido with your practitioner. If you need to treat the relationship, seek counseling. Schedule romantic dates with your loved one, exercise to increase your "feel good" hormones, enjoy an alcoholic beverage to loosen up (in moderation), try new routines in bed with your partner.

A healthy and active sex life is possible during and after menopause. See Chapter 7 for more information.

DEPRESSION

If you are suffering from hopelessness, apprehension and deep sadness for prolonged periods (two weeks or longer), you may be depressed. Do you feel worthless? Have you lost interest in your favorite activities? Are you angry? Have you felt hopeless? If you are suffering from lifestyle stress (change in relationship, financial reverses, loss of a loved one, caring for parents), seek support.

CAUSES: Depression is an illness that can be triggered by the chemicals in your brain. Serotonin regulates your moods. It is the "feel good" hormone. When serotonin levels drop due to fluctuating hormones, you can experience extreme episodes of depression. Some medications can worsen depression. It is important to review your medications with your practitioner.

SOLUTIONS: There is hope—hormone therapy, antidepressants and psychotherapy can help you if you are suffering from depression. If you have a history of clinical depression, be sure to discuss this with your practitioner. For more information, see Chapter 6.

ANXIETY

Feeling wound up, as if you may explode at any minute? Mild intermittent anxiety sometimes occurs during the menopausal transition. Generally these symptoms will subside over time.

CAUSES: Going through physical, emotional and midlife lifestyle changes can cause anxiety.

SOLUTIONS: Discuss your anxiety with your loved ones and friends; support can make a difference during anxiety attacks. If your anxiety seems out of control, discuss this with your health-care provider.

Once you understand your body's changes, it will be easier to manage menopause. Identifying your personal symptoms is the first step in creating a plan that fits your lifestyle.

Now that you know about menopause, why it happens, the stages and how it affects your life, you may be asking, "What do I do about it?" This is where the fun begins. *The Menopause Makeover* has an 8-Step, 12-Week Program that will give you the tools to do something about "it"!

chapter 2

Step One: Okay, So I'm Menopausal …
Now What Do I Do?
Understanding Your Treatment Options

Once you know that you are perimenopausal or meno-pausal, you're probably wondering, "So what can I do to feel better?" With numerous medical studies on hor-mone therapy and an abundance of purported remedies, making the correct choice can be difficult.

When I stopped taking birth control pills, I slammed into menopause, riddled with severe symptoms. I tried doing nothing, hoping I could tolerate these meno-pausal changes, but without success. Then I opted for some popular herbal remedies, whose properties for overcoming menopausal symptoms I now know are scientifically unfounded. Not surprisingly, I had no success. Next, I attempted visualization exercises, hoping that "seeing" a life free of hot flashes would help. That did not work. I even prayed nightly, asking God to "Please relieve my hot flashes!" God was listening, because I finally got it right. By combining hormone therapy (HT), complementary remedies (yoga and carefully selected supplements), as well as developing new exercise routines and committing to a new eating plan, I started feeling better. It took a combination of treatment options to regain control of my health and well-being. It took hard work. The payoff was the renewal of a happy and healthy me.

We are all different. No two of us have the same history, genetics, beliefs or comfort zones. Because there is no one formula, no magic pill, it can be challenging to treat menopause symptoms. If you have a family history of osteoporosis, heart disease or cancer, your treatment choices are critical to your health. It is important for you to take an active interest in managing your menopause, incorporating your personal beliefs, your genetic history and your current medical concerns. Because we have choices, we can find solutions.

The first step to creating a menopause management plan is to understand your treatment options.

OPTIONS FOR TREATING MENOPAUSE

- Lifestyle changes, such as diet and exercise
- Hormone therapy
- Complementary and Alternative Medicine (CAM)
- A combination of the above

LIFESTYLE CHANGES

Studies have clearly shown that good lifestyle habits, such as proper nutrition and regular exercise, can benefit your overall health. Being committed to good health, including no smoking and limited alcohol consumption, will give you more energy and help you sleep better. In addition, your mood and general outlook often improve. While there have been no formal studies confirming that diet and exercise alleviate menopausal symptoms, I can definitely report that I felt better after I lost weight and incorporated exercise into my daily routine. My high blood pressure went down and I enjoyed shopping for new clothes as a reward for my victories. Practicing healthy lifestyle habits is important during this phase of your life. The habits you establish now could add years to your life. There is more information about nutrition in Chapter 3 and about exercise in Chapter 4.

HORMONE THERAPY

If you have severe menopausal symptoms, you may be a good candidate for hormone therapy (HT). Hormone therapy is used to supplement the body with estrogen when the ovaries no longer produce adequate levels of the hormone and can help alleviate many of your symptoms, including hot flashes, vaginal dryness and night sweats. Hormone therapy can also reduce the risk of osteoporosis, lower the risk of colon cancer, and may reduce your risk for coronary disease, although this last point is controversial.

Since estrogen alone has been found to increase the risk of uterine cancer, most HT consists of progesterone, along with estrogen, which eliminates that cancer risk. If a woman has had a hysterectomy, and thus does not have a uterus, she does not need to take progesterone and can take estrogen by itself.

While hormone therapy can reduce the risk of some disorders or diseases (colon cancer, osteoporosis, vaginal atrophy), it can also increase the risk of others, such as breast cancer and blood clots. If you are at risk for breast cancer, blood clots or uterine (endometrial) cancer, discuss these issues with your doctor before starting hormone therapy.

Hormone therapy may seem intimidating at first, but it's really not that complicated—all you need to do is understand your options to decide what's right for you. At first, when discussing hormone therapy with my doctor, I was intrigued by transdermal application and bioidenticals. After trying this choice, I found that I did not actually like wearing a patch or applying creams. I preferred taking a pill, and I was a good candidate, so I take a pill every morning. Once you learn the basics, you will be able to discuss your preferences with your health-care provider. Let's get started!

WHAT TYPE OF HORMONE THERAPY IS RIGHT FOR YOU?

All women are different. Your medical history and genetics make you unique. Treating menopause symptoms and long-term health is very personal for each woman. When discussing hormone therapy, there are two basic options: estrogen therapy (ET) and estrogen plus progestogen therapy (EPT). The term *hormone therapy* (HT) covers both ET and EPT. The FDA refers to EPT as HT.

HORMONE THERAPY TERMINOLOGY

Estrogen therapy (ET): Estrogen alone, or "unopposed" estrogen, is prescribed for postmenopausal women who have had a hysterectomy. This is because, without a uterus, the risk of uterine cancer is essentially absent, so there is no need for the uterine protection of progesterone.

Estrogen plus progestogen therapy (EPT): A combination of both estrogen and progestogen (either progesterone or progestin—synthetic forms of progesterone). Progesterone, coupled with estrogen, eliminates the risk of uterine cancer by preventing stimulation of the uterine lining.

WAYS TO TAKE HORMONE THERAPY

Hormone therapy can be administered vaginally (with vaginal creams, rings or suppositories), through the bloodstream (pills) or transdermally (through the skin).

WAYS HORMONE THERAPY CAN BE ADMINISTERED

- Oral—the most commonly used formulation
- Transdermal—patch, gel and spray
- Vaginal—creams, rings and tablets
- Intrauterine device (IUD)—progesterone only

Your choice of HT administration is personal. Do you prefer to take a pill once a day, put on a patch once or twice a week, apply daily gel or spray to your skin or administer estrogen vaginally? We are all different. Talk to your practitioner and let her know what you prefer.

There are new studies investigating the benefits of transdermal application, which provides the same relief from symptoms as pills, but is absorbed differently. When you take a pill, it is processed through the liver. Transdermal options are absorbed by the skin, and so bypass the liver. Also, transdermal options can be prescribed in lower doses than pills, because they don't have to be digested.

If you are only suffering from vaginal symptoms (dryness or painful intercourse), vaginal application may be a good choice for you. The estrogen is delivered vaginally via creams or vaginal tablets (suppositories). You do not need to oppose the estrogen cream with progesterone, because the dose is so small that the only area treated is the vagina, and the cream is not absorbed significantly into your bloodstream. Vaginal HT application does not treat hot flashes and other menopause symptoms, just vaginal dryness.

Once you decide on your hormone recipe (ET or EPT), how you wish to take it (orally, transdermally or vaginally) and when you take it, your practitioner can prescribe the appropriate therapy, based on your needs and preferences.

TYPES OF HORMONES

In order to choose the right HT, it helps to understand the different types of hormones: how they are derived, how they are made and where. As I explain the different types of hormones, I'll clarify some of those confusing buzzwords for you—*natural, bioidenticals* and *compounding.*

The ingredients

In general, estrogen products are chemically synthesized, primarily from an active ingredient called diosgenin, a molecule extracted from the tubers and flowers of various plants including Dioscorea, a wild yam. Another source that is used to make conjugated estrogen, as is found in Premarin, is isolated from the urine of pregnant mares. These sources are then synthesized—altered through biosynthetic manufacturing processes—to create a formulation that can be used to produce the actual pills, patches, creams, gels or vaginal tablets.

Many of us want to use a "natural" product, since going through menopause is a natural transition. But you may be asking yourself, "How can the end product be 'natural' after it has been synthesized?" Sadly, the word *natural* is merely a marketing term. Some companies market their hormones as "natural" because the hormone they used had a plant origin. However, all hormones, whether made in compounding pharmacies or in manufacturers' laboratories, are synthetic in the sense that they are made by chemical processes.

After the 2002 Women's Health Initiative (WHI) results (increase in breast cancer, heart attacks and strokes), many of us were afraid to use hormone therapy, thinking it was harmful. That is when the word *natural* started being used to advertise hormones. *Natural* does not necessarily mean healthier and is primarily used for its advertising appeal.

How it is made

BIOIDENTICAL: A hormone manufactured in a laboratory that is chemically identical to the hormones produced by a woman's body. Bioidenticals are made of chemically altered ingredients from plant sources. Some believe a bioidentical hormone is a more "natural" option because it has the same molecular structure as our hormones, but the actual ingredients used in bioidenticals are synthesized (altered through chemical manufacturing processes) in a laboratory.

NONBIOIDENTICAL: A hormone manufactured in a laboratory that is not exactly chemically identical to the hormones produced by a woman's body. Nonbioidenticals also use synthesized ingredients derived from plant or animal sources.

Where are they made?

LABORATORY: A manufacturer's laboratory must abide by the FDA's rules and regulations. A hormone formulation created in a lab must follow FDA quality control on dosing and effectiveness. The ingredients and the process are FDA-approved. That means a lot of testing was done to make sure the treatment is safe for you. Your doctor can prescribe bioidentical HT produced in a regulated laboratory. Hormone products produced in a laboratory are also referred to as "conventional" therapy. Both bioidentical and nonbioidentical hormone therapies are produced in regulated manufacturers' laboratories.

COMPOUNDING PHARMACY: Compounding pharmacies combine, mix or alter ingredients to create a customized hormone for an individual patient. Unlike hormones that are made in a laboratory, compounding pharmacies have not demonstrated the safety, effectiveness and quality control, based on large, scientific studies, that the FDA requires of pharmaceutical manufacturers. Compounding pharmacies use chemically synthesized hormones made from plants—the same government-approved ingredients that are used in a manufacturer's laboratory. However, compounded "individualized" formulations are not necessarily uniform when it comes to purity, potency or efficiency. There is no registry of adverse effects from compounded medicines and there is no formal way to monitor adverse reactions.

A compounded formulation may benefit an individual who does not respond to conventional HT, or needs greater dosing flexibility, needs to avoid allergens or needs treatment options where there is no commercial product available (such as testosterone). Compounding pharmacies are regulated by state pharmacy boards using U.S. Pharmacopeia (USP) standards—the official public standard-setting authority for all prescriptions and over-the-counter medicines and dietary supplements—not federal FDA regulations.

Many women find compounded hormones appealing because they are marketed as a more "natural" option, but the ingredients are still the same synthesized hormones. I tried a common custom-compounded estrogen and my estrogen levels went through the roof. When I had a hormone blood test, my estrogen levels were almost seven times higher than normal! I suspect the mixtures were inconsistent, and I was probably not giving myself the exact doses every day. Using compounded hormones, made by your pharmacist and applied by you, leaves room for error. Mixing and application mistakes can dramatically affect you and your treatment results.

COMPOUNDING PHARMACY VERSUS LABORATORY

To better understand the differences, let's compare hormones that are made in a compounding pharmacy to conventional hormone therapy:

Compounding Pharmacy (bioidentical)	Conventional Laboratory (bioidentical and nonbioidentical)
Chemically identical to human hormones	Chemically identical or similar to human hormones
Lack of FDA oversight	Has FDA oversight
Unmonitored doses; may be inaccurate and may be inconsistent	Monitored doses; accurate and consistent
Not FDA-tested; unknown risks	FDA-tested; known risks
Effectiveness unproven	Effectiveness tested and proven
Insufficient scientific evidence	Scientific evidence exists, and is conclusive

Source: The Endocrine Society. Bioidentical Hormones Position Statement. October 2006. Available at: endo-society.org.

HORMONE THERAPY FACTS

Ladies, these are the facts:

1. Compounding pharmacies and manufacturers' laboratories use the same ingredients.

2. There is no scientific evidence that custom-compounded bioidenticals are safer or more effective than standard pharmaceutical bioidentical prescriptions. There are no large, placebo-controlled studies to support claims of their safety or effectiveness.

3. There are several standard prescription formulations of bioidentical estradiol and micronized progesterone that are FDA-tested and -approved. This type of prescription hormone therapy has been carefully standardized when it is manufactured. There are many standard FDA- approved bioidenticals available.

4. According to the FDA, roughly 30 million HT prescriptions per year are prepared in compounding pharmacies that are not regulated by the FDA.

5. Both the compounding pharmacies and the pharmaceutical companies promote their products. Bioidentical hormone therapy has provided the largest revenue stream of any compounded therapeutic drug category for the peri- and postmenopausal demographic.

6. Compounded bioidentical hormone therapy products do not have a "package insert" specifying risks or effectiveness, and they are not approved by the FDA.

7. An FDA survey (Center for Drug Evaluation and Research) ordered 29 products (various therapeutic uses and hormone therapies) from 12 compounding pharmacies and tested them. Thirty-four percent of these products failed at least one standard quality control test. Twenty-five percent failed potency standards among compounded hormones. When the FDA tested 3,000 pharmaceutical products, there was a failure rate of less than 2 percent for all tests.

So what does this all mean for you? Both compounding pharmacies and manufacturers' laboratories are essentially using the same ingredients. When choosing the hormone therapy that's right for you, keep in mind that both compounding pharmacies and pharmaceutical companies are in the business of making money—the word *natural* is a marketing term. Pharmaceutical companies must abide by strict FDA regulations to guarantee that your hormone products are safe and uniform, and the products were tested so you know your risks. Compounding pharmacies do not have the same restrictions.

DECIDING WHICH HORMONE THERAPY IS RIGHT FOR YOU

Your clinician will assess your individual situation and prescribe the hormone therapy she thinks will best address your symptoms or health concerns. Understanding your hormone options helps you participate in that choice and find the approach that's right for you.

No single hormone recipe will work for every woman. You must take the time to work with your health-care practitioner to make adjustments. During one of our many conversations on hormone therapy, Dr. Klein said, "You cannot give every woman the same dress—she has to try it on to see if it fits. Sometimes you have to alter the dress, so it fits better." This same philosophy applies to hormone therapy, as it does to many medications. You start out with the lowest dose, and make adjustments if necessary. The exception to this rule is the woman who is in abrupt surgical menopause, in which case, it is generally necessary to start with the higher dose of HT, and taper down as tolerated.

MENOPAUSE MAKEOVER
HORMONE THERAPY CHEAT SHEET

1. The only "natural" hormones are the hormones being made by your body.

2. Laboratories create molecules that are either identical (bioidentical) or not (nonbioidentical) to those in your body.

3. You have the choice of using a product that is regulated and tested or not.

4. Choose the product that works best for you. This may mean trying different doses or schedules or types until you find the right one.

5. Being informed is your first step to managing your menopause transition.

Review your symptoms and discuss your lifestyle with your doctor, so that you make the correct choices. If you decide that hormone therapy is the best option for you, understand what you are taking, the side effects and the risks.

COMMON SIDE EFFECTS OF HT

HT can help you feel more like yourself again, but there are potential side effects that you should be aware of.

UTERINE BLEEDING, OR SPOTTING: If you experience this, you can try a lower estrogen dose. Most bleeding from hormone therapy subsides over time. Unexpected, unusually heavy or recurring bleeding needs to be evaluated by your health-care provider.

BREAST TENDERNESS: Try a lower estrogen dose; switch to another estrogen; limit salt intake; switch to another progestin; limit caffeine and chocolate. Generally, after three months it subsides once you are on an established hormone regimen.

NAUSEA: Nausea is uncommon but usually subsides once you're on an established regimen.

BLOATING: Try switching to low-dose, non-oral estrogen, lowering the progesterone dose to a level that still protects the uterus.

FLUID RETENTION: Limit salt intake.

HEADACHE/MIGRAINE: Switch to non-oral estrogen; lower the dose of estrogen and/or progesterone; switch to a continuous-combined regimen; switch to progesterone or a 19-norpregnane derivative; drink water; limit intake of salt, caffeine and alcohol.

MOOD CHANGES WITH EPT: Make sure you are not suffering from depression or anxiety; lower the progesterone dose; switch progesterone; change to a continuous-combined EPT regimen.

CORNEA SHAPE CHANGES: Unfortunately, no current solution strategy exists. Good news—weight gain is *not* a
side effect of hormone therapy!

IS HORMONE THERAPY SAFE?

There is a lot of confusion regarding the safety of HT.
We have all seen the headlines and watched the news reports stating that hormone therapy has risks. Before the
2002 Women's Health Initiative (WHI) report, many
doctors treated menopausal women with HT, thinking the use of estrogen and progestin after menopause
helped protect women against heart disease. But in
2002, the WHI came out with a study that found an
increased risk of heart attack, stroke and breast cancer
for women postmenopause. Headlines warned women
against taking hormone therapy without fully disclos-
ing all the facts and issues pertaining to this study. The
HT public fear factor was so great that 56 percent of HT
users aged 50 and older tried to discontinue therapy
after this study. What was not revealed in those headlines was that the WHI was not studying treatment of
menopausal symptoms. It was a study focused on determining whether HT prevented chronic illnesses. The
average age of the participants was 63, with two-thirds
of them starting hormone therapy more than ten years
after menopause. Women with severe symptoms were
generally not included in the WHI. A few years later,
the WHI narrowed its focus on a second trial, looking
at the health effects of hormone therapy in younger
(under 60 years old) versus older women. They found

that younger postmenopausal women actually experienced a *lower* risk of adverse health effects from hormone therapy than their older counterparts.

There have been many other studies focusing on HT and heart disease, revealing that menopausal women between the ages of 50 and 59 who took HT for less than 10 years did not have an increased risk of heart disease. Women who began HT long after menopause did have an increased risk of adverse effects.

Hormone therapy is still the most effective treatment for menopausal symptoms. Discuss your concerns with your practitioner, who can help you decide whether to take hormone therapy, and, if so, at what age, the dosage and for how long.

HORMONE THERAPY AND CANCER

Will hormone therapy increase your risk of cancer? The good news is that, if taken in proper doses for a limited period (less than 5 years), HT has not been reported to increase your risk of breast and uterine cancers. HT does not typically affect cervical, ovarian or lung cancer risk, especially when used for less than five years. Results from the WHI study found that women on HT had a lower risk of colon cancer.

Throughout the past decade, research has consistently shown that HT only poses a risk if taken for longer than 5 years or in high doses. The risk appears to be greater with combined estrogen and progestin regimens than with estrogen alone. Be sure to talk to your doctor about whether HT is safe for you, as the degree of risk is based on personal history, family history and multiple other factors and must be evaluated on an individual, case-by-case basis.

Estrogen therapy (ET) and estrogen with progesterone therapy (EPT) can be powerful tools in managing menopause—they help relieve many symptoms. Since hormone therapy is prescribed at lower doses than in the past, it has fewer side effects. It is essential for each woman to weigh the individual benefits and risks of treatment. I personally found relief with hormone therapy. It also took a healthy eating plan, exercising most days of the week and incorporating yoga (a complementary remedy) into my life to feel normal again.

IF HORMONE THERAPY IS NOT AN OPTION

Hormone therapy isn't always an option. If you're at risk for breast cancer, heart disease, uterine cancer, stroke or deep vein thrombosis, or if you have a history of blood clotting, your clinician may advise you to consider other treatment options. Not to worry: You still have choices for treating symptoms.

COMPLEMENTARY AND ALTERNATIVE REMEDIES

Most of us would love to treat our menopause symptoms "naturally," since menopause is a "natural" event in our life. This involves using practices like yoga and acupuncture and products, such as herbs or phytoestrogens, that are not used by conventional

ALTERNATIVES TO HORMONE THERAPY

{ Medication options }

- Gabapentin (used for neurological purposes, to prevent seizures and for chronic pain syndrome) may be used to treat hot flashes, particularly for those occurring at night and disturbing sleep

- Antidepressants to treat irritability and hot flashes

- Clonidine (blood pressure medication) is sometimes used to treat hot flashes; possible side effects are dry mouth and sleep disturbances

{ Lifestyle options }

- Cardiovascular exercise 5–6 days a week

- Strength training 2–3 days a week

- Follow Menopause Makeover Food Pyramid (see page 91)

- No smoking

- Limited alcohol consumption

- Monitor blood pressure and cholesterol levels

- Layered clothing

{ Alternative and Complementary options }

- Calcium and vitamin D for bone health

- Black cohosh (Remifemin is a popular standardized brand) used to treat hot flashes and night sweats (more information on herbal remedies on page 48)

- Astroglide to treat vaginal dryness

- Practice relaxation techniques to manage hot flashes, sleep problems and moodiness (more on page 54)

medical practitioners. Complementary and Alternative
Medicine (CAM) incorporates a variety of healing phi-
losophies, therapies and approaches not conventionally
used by the Western medical community. A treatment
or remedy is *complementary* when it is used with *conventional* (mainstream medical community) therapies.
Alternative remedies are used instead of conventional
treatment. According to the National Institutes of
Health (NIH), over 36 percent of Americans use some
form of CAM. If you decide to use CAM to treat your
menopause symptoms, you're not alone.

PHYTOESTROGENS AND HERBAL TREATMENTS

Women have used herbs to treat menopause symptoms
for years. If you are going to use herbal remedies, be
sure to use products manufactured by reputable firms
to avoid unregulated production standards or contami-
nation. Alternative remedies do not have the U.S. Food
and Drug Administration's (FDA) stamp of approval
and are not usually covered by insurance. Scientific
tests or trials on many alternative products, such as
herbs, may not exist. Also be aware that long-term safety
data is lacking when it comes to herbal products.

The National Center for Complementary and
Alternative Medicine (NCCAM) at the NIH stimulates,
develops and supports research on CAM. In Canada,
CAM products are regulated by the National Health
Products Directorate (NHPD). NCCAM and NHPD

Web-site information can be found in the Resource Helpful Web sites section at the back of this book.

If your symptoms are mild and you choose CAM therapies to treat your symptoms, work closely with a health-care practitioner to ensure your safety. Many of these therapies are controversial. It is important to discuss all "natural" remedies with your doctor, as some herbal products can be dangerous if they are taken with other drugs. CAM therapies may not treat severe menopause symptoms and cannot treat osteoporosis and other diseases.

Phytoestrogens

INFORMATION: Phytoestrogens are plant-derived compounds with estrogen-like biological activity and a chemical structure similar to estradiol. You can find phytoestrogens in isoflavones (soybeans and soy products) and lignans (flax seed). Soy is also a wonderful source of protein and omega-3 fatty acids; it contains calcium as well. Soybeans, soy flour, miso soup, tempeh, tofu, tofu yogurt, soy hot dogs, soy milk and soy sauce all contain isoflavone. Apples, basil, barley, green tea, garlic, licorice, corn, parsley and sesame seeds also contain phytoestrogens.

USES: Many women use phytoestrogens to relieve menopausal symptoms, such as hot flashes, night sweats and vaginal dryness, and to improve cognitive function. Evidence regarding their effectiveness in treating hot flashes is mixed.

WARNINGS: Not every woman's body can convert soy iso-flavones into the plant-derived form of estrogen. Soy's possible role in breast cancer is uncertain. If you are at risk of developing breast cancer or other hormone-sensitive conditions (including ovarian or uterine cancer), discuss this with your practitioner.

Black Cohosh

INFORMATION: One of the most popular herbal treatments for menopause is black cohosh, because many believe it has estrogen-like properties. But recent research suggests that black cohosh acts more like a SERM (selective estrogen receptor modulator compounds that bind with estrogen receptors, exhibiting estrogen-like action in some tissues and anti-estrogenic action in other tissues) than an estrogen. Recently, the FDA required cautionary statements on packaging due to some reports of liver toxicity from excessive black cohosh use.

USES: Many women take this herb to treat hot flashes, night sweats, vaginal dryness, stress, arthritis and muscle pain. Studies of its effectiveness in reducing hot flashes have yielded mixed results, despite claims that women get hot-flash relief from black cohosh.

SIDE EFFECTS: Include gastrointestinal discomfort, headaches, nausea, vomiting and dizziness.

WARNINGS: Black cohosh has salicylate in it, so do not take it if you are taking aspirin or other blood thinners.

Chasteberry

INFORMATION: Also known as monk's pepper and sage tree hemp, chasteberry was used in the Middle Ages to decrease sexual desire.

USES: Women have reported improvements in mood, headaches and breast tenderness, but scientific evidence is lacking.

SIDE EFFECTS: Include GI problems, acnelike rashes and dizziness.

WARNINGS: Chasteberry may affect certain hormone levels. Do not take chasteberry if you are taking birth control pills. Chasteberry may also affect the dopamine system in the brain, so avoid it if you are using amantadine, levodopa, or SSRIs ("selective serotonin reuptake inhibitors," a class of antidepressants).

Valerian Root

INFORMATION: Valerian root was historically used to treat insomnia.

USES: A sleep aid, and to treat nervousness, depression, headaches, irregular heartbeat and anxiety. Valerian improves sleep when taken nightly for one to two weeks.

SIDE EFFECTS: Include headaches, dizziness, upset stomach and tiredness the morning after use.

WARNINGS: Valerian root can give you a hangover feeling, so use with caution.

Dong Quai

INFORMATION: Also known as tang gui.

USES: A blood thinner, and to treat hot flashes and cramps.

WARNINGS: Although taken to reduce hot flashes, studies found it was no better than a placebo. Dong quai contains compounds that can thin the blood, and it makes the skin more sensitive to the sun, so beware that this herb can be potentially toxic. Women with fibroids, hemophilia or other blood-clotting problems should not use dong quai.

Ginseng

INFORMATION: American ginseng is similar to Asian ginseng, *Panax ginseng, L.,* which grows wild in northern Manchuria.

USES: Relieves stress, mood symptoms and sleep disturbances; can stimulate a low sex drive and boost immunity. Ginseng has not been found to be helpful for the treatment of hot flashes. Some claim it can lower blood glucose and control blood pressure.

SIDE EFFECTS: Include nervousness, insomnia, headaches, GI problems, dizziness and hypertension, and can cause allergic reaction. Asian ginseng may lower levels of blood sugar. So if you have diabetes, use caution.

WARNINGS: Ginseng has been found to inhibit platelet aggregation (blood clotting). Do not combine with an anticoagulant, aspirin or vitamin E.

Ginkgo Biloba

INFORMATION: A blood thinner and antioxidant.

USES: Has been used to improve memory and promote a sense of well-being, although recent studies suggest that the use of ginkgo biloba does not improve memory.

SIDE EFFECTS: Include headache, GI distress, diarrhea, dizziness or allergic skin reactions.

WARNINGS: Do not combine with an anticoagulant, aspirin or vitamin E.

Red Clover

INFORMATION: Contains estrogen-like compounds.

USES: It is purported to decrease menopausal symptoms (hot flashes, vaginal dryness, mood swings), high cholesterol and osteoporosis, but scientific evidence is lacking. Some women claim that red clover can reduce hot flashes, but scientific evidence is lacking.

SIDE EFFECTS: Studies report few side effects and no serious health problems.

St. John's Wort

INFORMATION: Some say the name *St. John's Wort* refers to John the Baptist, as the plant blooms around the time of the feast of St. John the Baptist in late June.

USES: A popular treatment for anxiety, sleep disorders, mild to moderate depression and nerve pain. Some women take St. John's Wort together with black cohosh to relieve hot flashes, but scientific evidence is lacking.

SIDE EFFECTS: Dry mouth, GI upset, headache, dizziness, nausea, fatigue and sexual dysfunction.

WARNINGS: St. John's Wort has significant drug interactions, so it is important to discuss this herb's use with your health-care provider. Do not take St. John's Wort with SSRIs, birth control pills, or warfarin (a blood thinner). Take with food to avoid stomach upset. St. John's Wort may cause increased sensitivity to sunlight.

ALTERNATIVE PRACTICES

Alternative practices are often used to help alleviate menopausal symptoms. Many women find that they help, although, according to the National Center for Complementary and Alternative Medicine, continued research is needed to determine their effectiveness. At this time, there is not enough strong scientific evidence to recommend the use of herbs, according to NCCAM, the think tank at the NIH.

ACUPUNCTURE: Traditional Chinese Medicine (TCM) corrects energy imbalances using needles properly placed in various parts of your body. Some women claim they get relief from menopausal symptoms from acupressure and/or acupuncture. Because needles are used to perform acupuncture, hire a qualified specialist.

MASSAGE: Oriental massage is used to bring the body back into harmony. This is one of my favorite alternative practices.

YOGA: Yoga is a wonderful activity to add to your exercise and stress-management plan.

It helps to relieve stress, prevent osteoporosis, reduce mood swings, increase strength and flexibility, and improve self-esteem.

MEDITATION AND BREATHING EXERCISES: Believed to help calm the mind and body, resulting in self-acceptance and a sense of well-being.

AYURVEDA: India's traditional system of medicine, emphasizing balance between the mind, body and spirit to achieve harmony. Treatments include exercise, diet, meditation, massage, herbs and controlled breathing.

MIND-BODY MEDICINE: Hypnosis, biofeedback, music, dance, prayer, visual imagery, meditation and art therapy are all forms of mind-body medicine. Biofeedback has had some success controlling hot flashes and stress incontinence.

REFLEXOLOGY: The foot and sometimes the hand are massaged with pressure applied to *reflex* zones to restore proper balance and remove unhealthy blockages.

ENERGY MEDICINE: Reiki, gi gong and healing touch are therapies that focus on energy fields within the body or from outside sources.

COMBINATION OF TREATMENT OPTIONS

Be prepared to try a number of options before you have success. If you're like me, you will need to be patient and continue to search for the correct treatment option until you find one that works for you. Discuss your symptoms and treatment options with your health-care provider. Perhaps a combination of hormone therapy and complementary practices may bring you relief, as it did for me.

Remember, being informed is an asset during your menopause transition—keep up-to-date on the latest research and keep track of your symptoms over time.

As your symptoms change, you will most likely need to adjust your approach.

MAKEOVER TIPS

- Surround yourself with loved ones who support you.
- Become informed.
- Make lifestyle changes.
- Develop a partnership with your doctor or health-care practitioner.
- Document your symptoms.
- If you choose to use hormone therapy, it should be based on your individual needs and medical history.

MAKEOVER TAKE-ACTION LIST

- Document your symptoms (intensity and date) in your Symptoms Checklist on page 15 in Chapter 1.
- Visit your health-care provider and request an FSH blood test. Prepare ahead of time with the "Making the Most of Your Doctor's Visit" tips on page 10.
- What type of treatment course have you chosen to discuss with your doctor? _____
- Record your course of action for managing menopause symptoms under *hormones* on page 309.

IN YOUR ESSENTIAL PLANNER

- Record your appointments (doctor or other health-care practitioner, lab tests, medical tests) in your Month-at-a-Glance Planner.
- Record your hormone treatment and dosage each day (prescription or nonprescription) in your 12-Week Plan.
- Record any other medications you may be taking (blood pressure medication, cholesterol medication, antibiotics, aspirin, allergy medication) in your 12-Week Plan.
- Document your symptoms daily in your 12-Week Plan (hot flashes, night sweats, irregular periods, loss of libido). Do you see patterns in your symptoms?
- Record your emotional and physical concerns in your journal.
- How you feel each day is important. Note your feelings each day in your 12-Week Planner.

- Record your weekly progress, noting symptoms in your 12-Week Planner.
- Keep track of your support team in your Menopause Makeover Contacts.
- Complete the Menopause Makeover Medical Forms.

chapter 3

Step Two: Feeding the New You: How Food Can Set You Free!

Having always been one of the lucky ones who could eat anything without gaining a pound, I felt as if menopause tackled me from behind and tossed me into the air like a rag doll. I plummeted to earth, weighing an extra 25 pounds and measuring an additional 17 inches in less than six months!

I ran to the nearest bookstore and purchased diet books, ordered expensive premade diet food, called friends who were diet experts and subscribed to online diet programs—all to no avail. After months of failure, the only thing I had lost was control of my life.

Hopeless, I surrendered to my never-ending menopausal food cravings. Every afternoon, I sat in front of the television watching *Oprah,* eating a slab of Brie cheese, and nursing a bottle of red wine to numb my dismay at being so overweight. My poor fiancé witnessed his fun, sexy, independent bride-to-be fall into a hellish abyss of self-pity. Even his unconditional love and support could not save me when I was in this condition.

I have always been able to rescue myself, but

menopause pushed every dysfunctional button I had. I lost control over my body, my self-confidence and my life. I struggled with the fact that I was aging, and I could not stop it. I felt a sense of failure in my relationship with my future husband. I worried that I could no longer bear children, even though we didn't plan on having any. It became clear to me, or so I thought, that "the change" really meant "the end."

Those feelings added a hefty 25 pounds to my small frame in less than six months. I was living in a self-imposed "fat suit," hiding under baggy clothes, hoping no one would notice. My former self was screaming to get out.

Terrified that I would walk down the aisle looking like an overstuffed sausage, I made a startling discovery. My weight-loss goals were focused on the perception that I was not perfect. I thought I had to lose weight in order to find my perfect self again, as opposed to acknowledging that I was already perfect, just buried under a "fat suit." This fat suit was built on the fear of aging, hormonal cravings, midlife stress and far too many cookies, ice cream, cheese and wine. I was feeding an unhealthy body thousands of extra calories a day, fueling extra weight gain and unhappiness. Once I revised my goals so that I was feeding and nurturing the already perfect me that existed under my menopause fat suit, the perfect me reemerged! I did not have to search for my healthy weight. It already existed!

I started taking care of the perfect me, feeding her the food she needed to be healthy—and exercising.

Those extra 2,000 calories I was consuming daily while watching *Oprah* had produced a very impressive fat suit. (Note to Oprah: Your show gave me comfort; unfortunately so did the Brie cheese!)

Once I calculated the calories I needed to feed my healthy size, and redefined the food ratios I needed to consume, the zipper on the fat suit started unzipping. As motivation, I printed out copies of an "inspirational picture" of myself at my healthy weight—taken just two years earlier—that I placed on my desk and exercise machine. Three months later, and 25 pounds lighter, the healthy me emerged.

Eating the correct foods in the proper portions actually helped alleviate many of my miserable menopause symptoms. Food had set me free!

In this chapter, I will review important information regarding food so that you understand how to eat right for your changing body. Armed with the facts, you can set your weight-loss and nutrition goals in Part Two of the book and create a personal food plan to achieve those goals in Part Three.

A majority of women ages 45-55 will gain weight. During menopause, it is natural for the body to store some fat around your "middle," so that your waistline starts to disappear. It is normal to gain five to ten pounds during menopause, but it's really your *lifestyle* habits that cause you to gain weight. That's good news—it means that with small adjustments to your diet and exercise habits, you can outsmart menopause and keep your waistline trim!

Weight gain is often one of the most frustrating symptoms we experience during menopause. You may notice the fat around your hips, thighs and rear shifting upwards to your midsection. You may feel discouraged because weight-loss methods that worked before menopause no longer work. The good news is that five to ten pounds of weight gain during "the change" reflects a readjustment of your metabolism, and you can learn to live with this. However, beyond that, you are probably not being rigorous about watching your caloric intake or exercising sufficiently to balance your intake.

Going through so many changes during menopause will force you to look at your health, emotions and lifestyle choices. If you have gained an excessive amount of weight, understanding how your body is changing will give you the tools to manage your weight during menopause. Menopausal weight gain is a wake-up call to eat delicious, healthy food, and enjoy a more active lifestyle.

> Feed the healthy you.

WHY YOU GAIN WEIGHT DURING MENOPAUSE

A number of factors can contribute to that extra belly bulge during menopause.

THE PHYSICAL

TESTOSTERONE: Testosterone is a hormone produced by the ovaries and adrenal glands that is 50 to 60 percent lower by the time you go through menopause. When levels of testosterone decrease, your metabolism slows.

GENETICS: Look at your family tree. Do you have relatives who carry excessive weight around the abdomen? Genetics may also be a factor affecting weight gain.

SLOWER METABOLISM: Your metabolism slows as you age, so you cannot eat the same size portions as you did when you were younger. If you do, you will likely gain weight.

MEDICAL CONDITIONS: Medical conditions, such as insulin resistance (when your body becomes resistant to the insulin it produces) or an underactive thyroid, can cause weight gain; even certain medications can cause you to gain weight. Speak to your doctor if you think this is a possibility.

LIFESTYLE CHOICES

UNHEALTHY EATING: Many women with busy schedules do not have the time to prepare healthy meals with appropriate portions. Eating fast food, and comfort foods in large portions, will only contribute to weight gain.

NOT EXERCISING OR EXERCISING LESS: Most women taking care of a family, partner and parents are also balancing a career at the same time. It is understandable that making time to exercise takes a backseat to other priorities. During perimenopause through postmenopause, incorporating exercise into your daily routine is critical to staying healthy. (More on exercise in Chapter 4.)

TEN WAYS TO COPE WITH STRESS

1. Identify stress factors in your home life, work situation, schedule and lifestyle.

2. Relax. Spend 20 quiet minutes a day. Pray, meditate, do relaxation visualization exercises.

3. Communicate with loved ones. Ask for support.

4. Create a plan to resolve your stressful situations.

5. Incorporate exercise into your routine. Get physical. Plant a garden. Take daily walks.

6. Watch your food intake. Try to eat healthy foods and eliminate fast foods. Avoid excessive caffeine, alcohol and sugar, and absolutely avoid tobacco.

7. Focus attention on time management. Do essential tasks and prioritize other activities. Don't try to do everything at once.

8. Get enough sleep. Pamper yourself.

9. Take a vacation. Go somewhere you have always dreamed of going.

10. Decide to be happy, love yourself, laugh and remember that no one is perfect.

MEDICATIONS

PRESCRIPTION DRUGS: Some prescription drugs can contribute to weight gain. The most common culprits are antidepressants. If you started gaining weight after beginning a new prescription, discuss this with your health-care provider. Do not stop taking your medications without a conversation with your doctor or clinician.

THE EMOTIONAL EATER

Emotional eating is very common—many people eat when they feel sad, lonely or stressed. But you don't have to let emotional eating sabotage your Menopause Makeover! The first step to conquering emotional eating is awareness.

Are You an Emotional Eater?

Did your parents give you food as a reward when you were a child?

Are you frustrated with something in your life?

Are you bored with your life or someone in your life?

Are you sad about a situation in your life?

Are you lonely?

If you answered, "yes" to at least three of these questions, you may be an emotional eater. As women, we are emotional creatures. Many of us eat to find comfort. Living in a society where women have careers, families, homes and financial responsibilities—no wonder we are grabbing brownies and cupcakes!

STRESS: THE DIET SABOTEUR

When your body is under stress, the hormone cortisol tells your body to go into storage mode for survival. Your body thinks it is in trouble and starts storing calories, causing weight gain. Stress hormones may block weight loss. You can experience stress from daily emotional events, dieting, lack of sleep from night sweats and depression. If you have unresolved emotional issues, they may surface during your menopause transition. This type of cortisol-induced stress can lead to food cravings, overeating, a slower metabolism, fluctuating blood sugar levels and fat storage around the waistline. If you are struggling with weight issues, take a look at the levels of stress in your life.

HIDING UNDER A FAT SUIT

As we get older, we start noticing the effects of aging, we experience weight gain and many of us struggle with the reality that having children is no longer possible. For many, these changes can affect our self-esteem. When we don't feel good about ourselves, it is common for us to overeat, and stop taking care of our health in general—both physical and emotional. Often we start to feel "safe" hiding under a self-imposed fat suit.

One of the first steps to living your perfect weight is addressing unresolved emotional issues. When you commit intellectually and emotionally to living your perfect weight, the rest of the journey is the execution of your menopause weight-management plan.

Why are you hiding under a fat suit?

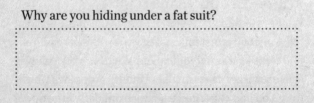

TEN WAYS TO CONQUER EMOTIONAL EATING

1. Identify what feelings come up for you when you reach for a pint of ice cream.

2. If you're bored, find an activity you can do when you feel emotional and start craving sugar, alcohol or salty foods. Take a walk, clean the house, work in your garden or call a friend.

3. When you feel emotional eating taking over during a stressful situation, close your eyes, breathe deeply and think of someone who loves you or whom you love. On every inhalation, breathe in *love;* on every exhalation, breathe out **stress.** Fill yourself with *love,* not ice cream.

4. Start a daily journal and record your feelings when you feel the urge to eat.

5. If you're overworked and feeling exhausted, remember to make time for yourself: Take a nap, make time to exercise or take a yoga class.

6. If you're lonely, find a buddy who also struggles with emotional eating and create a support team.

7. If you're anxious, think about why this might be. Are you are drinking too much coffee? Stressed at work? Identify the trigger and work to lessen the stress.

8. If feeling frustrated with a life situation or a particular person, confront it or him or her, and find a way to deal with the situation. Can you find a solution for the situation challenging you? If someone is driving you crazy, try to stand in the other person's shoes, be positive and create healthy boundaries. Instead of complaining about a situation or person, search for a life lesson to learn and then move on.

9. Remove tempting food from your house and office. This way you're more apt to eat when you're hungry, not emotional.

10. If emotional eating, stress, depression or anxiety becomes a larger issue, seek professional help.

There are many logical explanations for gaining weight during menopause. Whether physical, emotional or lifestyle choices, understanding the causes allows you to conquer and manage unwanted and un-healthy weight.

FOOD CAN SET YOU FREE

After you address any unresolved emotional issues that may be contributing to your weight gain, the next important factor in managing weight is learning how food can set you free. There are three categories of food: proteins, fats and carbohydrates. In order to maintain health, you need to consume nutrients from all three of these categories.

PROTEIN IS THE HERO

The word *protein* is derived from a Greek root meaning "of first importance." Your muscles, organs, bones, carti-lage, antibodies, skin, some hormones and all enzymes are made of protein.

Consuming the correct amount of protein has important benefits

1. Protein (chicken, turkey, beef, fish and beans) is processed more slowly from the stomach to the intestine. This makes you feel full longer. Protein does not stimulate the release of insulin, so it helps stabilize blood sugar.

2. Consuming protein low in saturated fat can improve your blood triglycerides and high-density lipopro-tein. This can reduce your risk of heart attack or stroke.

3. Protein is indispensable for the growth and maintenance of the cells in our body.

4. Our body development, healing of wounds, replacement of dead cells, hair and nail growth and the replenishment of lost blood is dependent on protein.

5. Proteins, in the form of enzymes, antibodies and hormones, can promote a strong, healthy metabolism and boost the nervous and immune systems.

Not consuming enough protein can lead to weakening of the muscles, heart and respiratory system; impaired growth; decreased immunity; and even death. As you go through menopause, protein is the hero—it helps keep your body from clinging to fat.

SOY IS A STAR

Soy is a wonderful source of protein. *Archives of Internal Medicine* found a link between soy consumption and strong bones. Women who consumed 13 grams a day of soy had a 35 to 37 percent lower risk of fractures compared to women in the lowest intake group. Soy also contains other wonderful nutrients, such as omega-3 fatty acids, fiber and B vitamins. If you do not consume meats or other animal products, soy protein is a healthy alternative. Both the American Dietetic Association and the Food and Drug Administration confirm that people who eat 25–50 grams of soy protein a day can help lower their levels of LDL cholesterol ("bad" cholesterol, which can clog blood vessels).

Other yummy nonmeat sources of protein are beans and legumes, nuts, peanut butter, cheese, whole grain products and yogurt.

COMPLETE VERSUS INCOMPLETE PROTEINS

Not all proteins are created equal. Proteins from animal sources (meat, fish, poultry, milk, cheese and eggs) are *complete proteins*. They contain all nine essential amino acids for human use. The only exception is soy (a plant source); it is also considered a complete protein. Amino acids are the chemical building blocks from which new proteins are made. Consuming complete proteins is important. Proteins obtained from plant-based foods (grains, cereals, legumes, seeds, nuts, lentils, peas and beans) are *incomplete proteins*. They do not possess the necessary amounts of essential amino acids for human use.

Why does this matter? If you are fulfilling a protein serving by consuming only nuts, it is not a *complete* protein. You need to have a variety of incomplete proteins to make up a complete protein. You can combine plant and animal foods, or plant proteins from a variety of grains and cereals for one meal or eat them separately at another meal to make up a complete daily protein serving.

HOW PROTEIN CAN BURN THAT BELLY FAT

For your Menopause Makeover, it's important to eat plenty of protein—a source of protein at every meal and snack. You should consume protein five to six times per day. The portion should be the size of the palm of your hand, around four to six ounces.

::

PERFECT PROTEINS FOR YOUR MENOPAUSE MAKEOVER

Choose Lean, Low-fat Protein Sources

Fish and Shellfish

- Flounder
- Salmon
- Cod
- Halibut
- Trout
- Crab
- Seabass
- Tuna (canned in water)
- Shrimp

Poultry

Remove the skin before cooking

- Chicken
- Turkey breast
- Ground chicken and turkey

Milk, Yogurt and Cheese

Skim or low-fat dairy can help keep bones strong.

- Cottage cheese
- Yogurt
- Fat-free milk

Low-fat cheeses:

- Swiss
- Ricotta
- Romano
- Mozzarella
- Farmer's cheeses
- Parmesan
- Jarlsberg
- Provolone
- Feta, Goat cheeses

Meat

- Ground beef
- Pork tenderloin
- Beef (lean cut)
- Sirloin steak

Eggs

You can eat egg whites daily—much lower in calories
and fat than if you include the yolks.

- Egg (medium)
- Egg whites

Legumes and Nuts

Legumes and nuts are loaded with fiber, helping you feel full for hours.

- Lima beans
- Almonds
- Lentils
- Cashews
- Walnuts

Soy

Soy protein can help lower cholesterol and reduce the risk of heart disease.

- Soybeans
- Tofu

Protein Snacks On-the-go

Great protein snacks include cereal bars,
energy bars, or meal-replacement drinks.

• • • **MENOPAUSE MAKEOVER PLANNER ENTRY** • • •

Go to the shopping list in the Essential Planner on page 357
and check off your favorite *healthy* protein choices.

FAT: THE GOOD, THE BAD AND THE UGLY

Fat, like protein, is vital to your health. In moderate
amounts fat transports oxygen to every cell in your
body. Fat is a component for building cells and body
tissue, and absorbing some vitamins and other nutrients. It is also an essential component in maintaining
hormones, the brain and the nervous system.

- Fat provides energy for your body to stay warm. Excess calories are stored in fat deposits that insulate the body.

- Fat helps protect your body from injury.

- Fat helps maintain healthy skin.

- Fats can help the body process proteins and carbohydrates.

- Eating food with fat can help us feel a sense of fullness.

- Fats regulate cholesterol metabolism.

- The texture of fat can make food taste creamy and smooth and carry flavor.

- Fat carries fat-soluble vitamins, such as vitamins A, D, E and K, by assisting in absorption from the intestines.

- Fat cushions our vital organs, like the kidneys.

- Consuming fat is important for normal brain development.

- Fat is a secondary source of energy.

Consuming the correct amount of fat has benefits
Consuming the correct type of fat, in the proper quantities, has some excellent benefits. There are three naturally occurring types of fats (monounsaturated, polyunsaturated and saturated), and one human-made fat (trans fat).

THE GOOD FATS
The good news is we can include good fats in our diet.

Monounsaturated Fats
The healthiest fat choice is monounsaturated fats. Olive oil, canola oil, peanut oil, macadamia oil, almonds, peanuts, pecans, cashews and avocados all contain mono–unsaturated fats. Vegetable oil fats remain liquid at

room temperature, and are one of the healthiest oils to add to your food plan. Monounsaturated fats can lower your bad cholesterol (LDL) levels, and increase your good cholesterol (HDL) levels. I want to repeat this because it is so important: Monounsaturated fats help increase good cholesterol and lower bad cholesterol! Stock your house with olive oil, almonds and avocados.

Polyunsaturated fats
Polyunsaturated fat is found in fish (salmon, halibut, herring and mackerel), soybeans, fish oils and grain products. This kind of fat is essential in our diet because polyunsaturated fat includes essential fatty acids—omega-3s and omega-6s—that our body cannot make for itself. Polyunsaturated fats can help lower the level of bad cholesterol (LDL).

Omega-3 fats can be found in fish oil. Polyunsaturated fish oils can protect the heart by lowering triglyceride levels and preventing blood clots. Natural sources of omega-3 fats are salmon, sardines, herring and rainbow trout.

If you are not a fish lover, you can also find omega-3s in flaxseed, canola and soy oils, plus flax seeds, soybeans, pumpkin seeds and walnuts.

Omega-6 fats can be found in soybean oil, corn oil, sunflower oil and cottonseed oil, and there are unproven claims that it is good for your skin and hair, and even that it promotes emotional health. However, omega-6 fats should be taken in moderation, because consuming high levels of omega-6 can interfere with the known health benefits of omega-3s. Recent studies suggest that higher levels of omega-6s may increase the risk of other diseases and can contribute to depression. Omega-6s, found in vegetable oils, may even contribute to an increased breast cancer risk in postmenopausal women.

Those following a typical Western diet consume a ratio of ten to one (10:1) of omega-6 to omega-3 fats, often as high as 30:1. This high level of omega-6 fats limits the health benefits of omega-3s. According to the National Institutes of Health and the U.S. National Library of Medicine, both omega-3 and omega-6 fats must work in balance to benefit your health. Aim for a 4:1 ratio or lower for optimum benefits.

THE BAD FATS
Just as there are good fats, there are bad fats. Bad fats include refined oils, partially hydrogenated oils, shortening and commercially deep-fried foods. Fat is a concentrated source of calories, so we must closely monitor our intake. A diet too high in fat is linked to higher risk of weight gain, high blood pressure, certain cancers and insulin resistance, as well as gallbladder disease.

Saturated fat
Saturated fat is found in red meat and other animal products, such as dairy products (including cheese, sour cream, ice cream and butter), lard and tropical oils, such as coconut oil and coconut milk, cocoa butter and palm oils. Saturated fats remain solid at room temperature.

Saturated fats raise LDL (bad) cholesterol, which can lead to hardening of the arteries, and they contribute to blood clots. Blood clots can lead to clogged blood vessels that can result in a stroke or a heart attack. When you purchase cheese, ice cream, sour cream and other dairy products, be sure to select low-fat options.

Trans fat

Trans fat is a human-made fat, created by adding hydrogen to a polyunsaturated fat; this turns liquid oils into more solid fats like margarine. Trans fats can be found in baked goods, fried foods, donuts, French fries, crackers and snacks. Trans fats raise your LDL (bad) cholesterol levels, lower HDL (good) cholesterol levels and increase your risk of heart disease. This is a double-whammy bad fat choice! The American Heart Association recommends an intake of no more than 1 percent of total trans fat calories per day.

THE UGLY

Since fat takes longer to digest than either protein or carbohydrates, you feel full longer after eating it. Yes, that fried chicken and bag of French fries will fill you up!

Many health organizations recommend a diet of no more than 30 percent fat per day. During menopause your body is clinging to fat. For your Menopause Makeover, I suggest a daily calorie intake of 25 percent fat, with the emphasis on *good* fats.

MAKEOVER TIPS

- Replace butter with olive oil.
- Consume leaner red meats: pork loin, pork tenderloin, extra-lean ground beef.
- Consume lean protein: chicken without the skin, turkey, fish.
- Broil, bake or grill meat. If you need to fry, use a nonstick pan with only a small amount of vegetable oil spray.

CHART OF GOOD FAT SOURCES

Olive oil	Macadamia oils	Mackerel	Almonds
Flaxseed	Peanut oil	Herring	Walnuts
Flaxseed oil	Rainbow trout	Sardines	Pecans
Canola oil	Salmon	Tuna	Cashews
Sunflower oil	Halibut	Avocado	Sunflower seeds
Safflower oil	Flounder	Olives	
Pumpkin oil	Crab, blue	Soybeans	
Soybean oil	Haddock	Peanuts	

• • • MENOPAUSE MAKEOVER PLANNER ENTRY • • •

Select healthy fat sources from this chart
and enter them in your "shopping list" on page 357.

THE TRUTH ABOUT CARBOHYDRATES

Carbohydrates are an important part of a healthy diet. Without any carbohydrates in your diet, you could feel fatigued, have muscle cramps and suffer from poor mental function. Who needs poor mental function when you are going through menopause?

Carbohydrates, also known as "carbs," provide the body with fuel for physical activities and for proper organ function. Your body breaks down carbs, and turns them into glucose. We often refer to glucose as blood sugar. As we get older, and experience the menopause transition, not all carbs are "friendly" to our food plan. Most carbohydrates provide comfort, so many of us grab comfort carbs when suffering with menopause symptoms. It is critical to make healthy carb choices during your menopause transition. Understanding the difference between "good" and "bad" carbs can be an important step in gaining control over your menopause symptoms, such as weight gain, and your overall health.

Consuming the *good* carbohydrates can:

- Provide easily obtained energy for your cells, tissues and organs.
- Provide essential vitamins and minerals.
- Provide an excellent source of fiber.
- Aid digestion and help your body reserve energy.
- Strengthen muscle tissue.
- Benefit blood sugar levels because good carbs break down slowly, so glucose is released gradually into your system.
- Improve mental concentration.
- Improve your mood.

Complex Carbohydrates

Complex carbs, commonly known as "starches," include whole-grain breads, cereals, brown rice, potatoes, starchy vegetables (corn, peas) and legumes (beans, lentils). Complex carbs take the body longer to digest because they are made up of chains of glucose molecules. The digestive system has to work harder to break down this chain into individual sugars so your body can absorb them. Since complex carbs take longer to digest, they give you energy that lasts longer. Complex carbs often provide fiber. Wonderful carbs that can also provide fiber are fruits, vegetables and whole grains; whole-grain bread; and whole-grain pastas and cereals. These are "friendly" carbs, if consumed in moderation.

Simple carbohydrates

Simple carbohydrates have smaller molecules of sugar, unlike the long chains of glucose found in complex carbs, and are digested quickly. Many products processed and prepared with refined sugar are simple carbs (white sugar, white pastas, white bread, cakes, chocolate, biscuits). These are not "friendly" carbs for gals struggling with menopausal weight gain and fluctuating hormones, because they are absorbed quickly, increasing the chances of the sugar being converted to fat. But fruits that are *natural* simple carbohydrates—those high in fiber, like apples, pears, oranges and strawberries—can actually help slow digestion, decreasing the surge of sugar energy into your cells when it's not needed, so your chance of converting it to fat decreases.

Other simple carbs are dairy products. Low-fat dairy products are healthy choices for your Menopause Makeover.

BLOOD SUGAR—THE UPS AND DOWNS

The Glycemic Index

Once we consume carbs, our body converts these carbs into energy very differently, depending on whether they are simple or complex carbs. Understanding this difference can help you conquer unwanted weight gain.

The Glycemic Index (GI) is a scale that ranks carbohydrate-rich foods based on how quickly and how high they boost blood sugar compared to pure glucose. The glycemic index number is the average amount that a particular food raises blood sugar levels. Eating high-glycemic foods (simple carbs) like white bread, soda, pasta dishes, and chocolate bars cause dramatic peaks in your blood sugar. Eating low-glycemic foods (complex carbs) like breakfast cereals (made of wheat bran, oats and/or barley), lentils, soybeans, baked beans and fruit causes a more gradual change in blood sugar. Eating low-glycemic foods can help you manage your weight, prevent insulin resistance and control type 2 diabetes.

Benefits of low-glycemic carbohydrates

- Low-glycemic carbs stabilize blood sugar levels in your body, and sustain those levels for longer periods.

- Your hunger urges are controlled because the blood sugar levels are released into your bloodstream more slowly.

- You are able to exercise for longer periods.

- Your risk of getting type 2 diabetes is lowered.

- Your risk of getting heart disease is lowered.

- Most low-glycemic foods are lower in calories and fat.

- Many low-glycemic foods are loaded with fiber and nutrients.

- Low-glycemic carbs can help you lose weight during menopause.

All carbohydrates are broken down into simple sugars during digestion. This activates the production of insulin in your pancreas. As blood sugar levels increase, cells in the pancreas create more insulin to absorb the blood sugar. When this happens, the sugar levels in your bloodstream start falling. Then your pancreas starts making a hormone called glucagones to signal the liver to start releasing stored sugar. When this process is working properly, your body and brain have healthy levels of blood sugar.

When the cells do not respond to the insulin signal to receive sugar, insulin resistance can occur. Insulin resistance causes your blood sugar and insulin levels to stay high long after eating, thus causing the production of insulin to slow down or even stop.

Insulin resistance can be dangerous to your health. It can increase your risk of type 2 diabetes, some cancers and heart disease.

Fortunately, cutting down on the consumption of refined grains, and/or replacing them in your diet with whole grains, plus consuming low-glycemic carbs, can decrease your chance of insulin resistance and help you achieve a healthy weight.

THE GI AND YOUR HORMONES

Your food choices can make a drastic difference in your menopause symptoms. Eating a high-glycemic diet can affect the way your hormones are metabolized by slowing the production of estrogen from the adrenal glands. This is the last thing you want when your estrogen is naturally declining! Ever-changing hormones and stressful midlife changes can affect the way your body regulates insulin. Eating low- to medium-glycemic foods can help regulate insulin. Maintaining balanced blood sugar levels can help limit overstimulation of the adrenals. You don't want your blood sugar and hormones both going haywire at the same time. Eating low- to medium-glycemic foods can help reduce mood swings, lower anxiety, improve your energy levels and help you succeed with your weight-loss plan.

Choose your carbs cautiously! Aim to consume low- to medium-glycemic carbohydrates.

LOW GLYCEMIC (55 OR LESS)	MEDIUM GLYCEMIC (56-69)	HIGH GLYCEMIC (70+)
Bran cereals	Brown rice	French fries
Legumes	Oatmeal	White potatoes
High-fiber fruits (apples, plums, oranges, cherries) and vegetables (broccoli)	Rice cakes	Candy bars
	Whole-grain breads	White rice
	Whole-grain pasta	White-flour pasta
Plain yogurt	Fruit juice without added sugar	Fruit juice with added sugar
Soy beverage	Pineapple	Sugar-sweetened beverages
All-bran	Bananas	Refined breakfast cereals
Oat bran	Raisins	
Sweet potato or yams	Popcorn	Watermelon
Fat-free milk	Split peas	Dried dates
	Couscous	Sugary snacks
	Shredded wheat cereal	Soda crackers
	Rye bread	Bagels, white
		Instant rice

• • • MENOPAUSE MAKEOVER PLANNER ENTRY • • •

Select healthy carbohydrate choices and enter them in your "shopping list" on page 358.

MAKEOVER TIPS

- ○ Consume low- to medium-glycemic foods.
- ○ Eat high-fiber complex carbs.
- ○ If you consume a high-glycemic food, combine it with low-GI food. For example, if you eat corn flakes for breakfast (high GI), add some strawberries (low GI) to make it a medium-glycemic value.
- ○ Include at least one low-glycemic choice for each meal.
- ○ Replace white bread with rye or oat-bran bread in your diet.
- ○ Fruits and vegetables are healthy carb choices during the menopause transition.

FIBER IS OUR FRIEND

Fiber is the part of plants that cannot be digested. All fruits, grains, vegetables and legumes contain fiber. Fiber is usually found in the outer layer of the plant, and is considered a carbohydrate. When you eat fiber, it passes through your body virtually unchanged.

Benefits of fiber

- ○ Helps keep your bowel movements regular and stools soft.
- ○ Moves fat through your digestive system more quickly—an added benefit in the battle against midsection belly fat.
- ○ Can help you lose weight.
- ○ Leaves you feeling full longer.
- ○ Keeps your blood sugar on an even keel.
- ○ Can help transport bad cholesterol out of your body.

- Can help reduce the risk of certain diseases (heart disease, diabetes).

Fiber is broken down into two categories—insoluble and soluble. Insoluble fiber cannot be dissolved in water. Soluble fiber can dissolve in water.

SOURCES OF FIBER

Soluble			
Apples	Beans	Nuts	Apple pulp
Strawberries	Lentils	Seeds	
Blueberries	Oatmeal	Rice bran	
Pears	Oat bran	Peas	
Insoluble			
Carrots	Whole-wheat breads	Whole-grain cereals	Brussels sprouts
Cucumbers			Cauliflower
Celery	Brown rice	Wheat bran	Beets
Tomatoes	Barley	Rye	
Zucchini	Couscous	Cabbage	

• • • MENOPAUSE MAKEOVER PLANNER ENTRY • • •

Add healthy fiber choices to your "shopping list" in the Essential Planner on page 358.

One of the primary benefits of *soluble fiber* is that it can lower blood cholesterol. And an excellent benefit of *insoluble fiber* is that it works as a laxative to move food along. You should consume 21 to 25 grams of fiber per day. Fiber is a wonderful part of your diet.

MAKEOVER TIPS

I

- Snack on raw vegetables and fruit when you get the munchies.
- Replace white pasta, breads and rice with whole-grain pasta, breads and rice.
- Incorporate a bowl of whole-grain cereal into your food plan for breakfast.

WATER

Two-thirds of our body weight is water. Blood is 83 percent water, muscles 75 percent, bone 22 percent and the brain 74 percent. So water is obviously good for you. Without water you would dehydrate, and your vital organs would shut down. Water is a necessity for life itself. Water is the most important molecule, second to oxygen, to live.

Benefits of drinking water

- Water keeps skin healthy and radiant.
- Water helps regulate body temperature.
- Water transports nutrients to your organs.
- Water removes waste.
- Water maintains overall health.

How much water do you need to consume?

There is no one water consumption formula that works for everyone. The Institute of Medicine advises that women consume 9 cups (2.2 liters) of total beverages per day.

YOUR PERSONAL WATER NEEDS
DEPEND ON MANY FACTORS:

• For every 20 minutes of exercise you do each day, drink 8 ounces of water.
• Hot or humid weather can increase sweating, increasing your fluid retention.
• If you are ill, suffering from a fever, vomiting or diarrhea causing a loss of fluids, drink more water. If you are suffering from kidney, liver or adrenal disease, discuss your water intake with your doctor.
• If you drink alcohol, add an equal amount of water. For example, 6 ounces of wine should be matched with 6 ounces of water consumption.
• Bottom line: hydrate based on your needs.

On average, 80% of your body's water comes from drinking water and beverage sources, and 20% of water comes from food sources. Many women consume coffee, tea and sodas, thinking they are sources of water. Although they are made mostly with water, nothing can replace the enormous benefits of pure water. Limit yourself to no more than two three-ounce cups of caffeinated beverages (coffee, tea, soda) per day. If you are on blood pressure medication, such as diuretics, or have a history of heart problems or swelling in your legs, you may need to adjust your fluid intake, so discuss this with your health-care provider!

LIMIT ALCOHOL

Too much alcohol can disrupt your sleep and trigger hot flashes. Lately there have been new reports claiming that minimal red wine consumption is good for you. It may be, but consume no more than 6 ounces per day. Remember, red wine has calories, too.

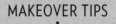

MAKEOVER TIPS

- Drink more water during exercise to replace water lost from sweating.

- If you don't like to drink water, enjoy fruits and vegetables that are high in water content (celery, tomatoes, oranges, melons).

- Drink sparkling water on ice with a twist of lemon.

- If you consume caffeinated drinks (coffee, tea, soda), alcohol drinks or salty foods, drink more water to avoid dehydration.

- It is generally a good idea to drink a glass (one cup) of water with every meal and a glass of water between each meal.

BEWARE OF SALT

Just as we cannot live without water, we cannot live without salt. When we cry, our tears are salty. When we sweat, our perspiration is salty. Salt can cure, seal, clean, preserve and act as an antiseptic. And salt is absolutely calorie-free.

So what *is* salt? It is a dietary mineral that is essential for human life. It is a mineral primarily composed of sodium chloride. The body needs a certain amount of sodium to function properly. The average adult stores approximately 250 grams of salt (that is about four salt shakers' worth of salt). We lose salt through normal body functions, so it is important to consume a healthy amount of salt daily. However, consuming too much salt is not beneficial. If you eat too much salt, your body may retain water, causing weight gain, increased blood pressure and hypertension, all of which increase your risk of stroke and heart disease.

Benefits of salt

- Helps the body absorb potassium.
- Helps maintain the correct concentration of body fluids.
- Crucial in transmitting electrical impulses through the nervous system.
- Helps cells absorb nutrients.
- Essential in ensuring that our muscles and nerves work properly.
- Helps maintain normal blood pressure.

The American Heart Association recommends consuming less than 2,300 milligrams (one teaspoon) of salt per day. Almost all processed foods—junk food, chips, bacon, cheese, pickles, fast food, meat products and breads—have high levels of salt. Recent studies reveal that 77 percent of a person's salt intake is from processed foods. Throw in the salt we add to food during preparation and eating, and most people are overconsuming salt.

The Center for Science in the Public Interest claims that excess salt is the single most harmful element in the food supply—even worse than saturated fat and trans fat, or food additives and pesticides! Salt is also a major cause of high blood pressure. During menopause, reducing salt from your diet will help alleviate fluid retention. Do not add salt to your food and reduce your overall salt intake by eating fewer processed foods and being mindful of your salt intake.

REASONS TO QUIT

If you are a smoker, now is a good time to stop. Smoking has been linked with early menopause, and oftentimes with the appearance of wrinkles earlier in life. More than 178,000 women die each year from smoking-related diseases. It is not too late to quit smoking. There are chewing gums, prescriptions, patches and support groups to help you quit. If you smoke, now is the time to quit.

MAKEOVER TIPS

- Don't add salt while cooking or at the table.
- Eat fresh foods—they do not have salt added.
- Season with herbs and spices, instead of salt (lemon, garlic, paprika).
- Avoid processed foods (frozen meals, fast foods, convenience foods and many canned foods).
- Use soy sauce sparingly (created by soaking soybeans in salt).
- Avoid bacon, sausage, ham, cheese, pizzas and stock cubes.
- Avoid salted chips, nuts, crackers or other salty snacks.

THE MENOPAUSE MAKEOVER FOOD PYRAMID

The USDA has food pyramid guides with the recommended food ratios for the general population. Dietary Approaches to Stop Hypertension (DASH) has a food pyramid for people suffering from high blood pressure. There are government food pyramids for folks over 70 and vegetarians. Yet there are no "official" government-recommended food guides for women going through menopause. Because a woman's body is changing, her food ratios must change as her body changes. In the past, the USDA recommended food ratios of 53 percent carbohydrates, 29 percent fat and 18 percent protein. This recommendation does not work for women going through "the change."

As your hormones begin to fluctuate, and fat starts clinging to your midsection, a diet promoting 53 percent carbohydrates won't help you stay trim during menopause! Plus, the USDA's plan lumps men and women into the same category—rubbish! We may be equal in most other ways, but we are not physically the same. Am I questioning the USDA? Absolutely! During my menopausal transition, I followed the USDA food ratio recommendations, and only gained weight and became more frustrated. Most diet plans, books and programs are based on the USDA food ratios. No wonder menopausal women are unhealthy and gaining weight.

There are no official government studies on what the correct eating ratios are for menopausal women; I had the task of exploring different ratios for myself.

What I discovered was that I had to increase my protein intake, and decrease my high-glycemic carbohydrate intake. The answer is the Menopause Makeover Food Pyramid—the key to eating well during menopause.

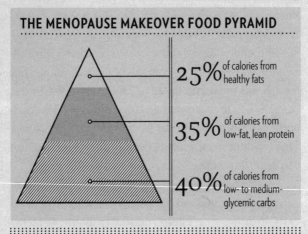

THE MENOPAUSE MAKEOVER FOOD PYRAMID

25% of calories from healthy fats

35% of calories from low-fat, lean protein

40% of calories from low- to medium-glycemic carbs

If you make this adjustment in your food ratios, you'll find that it's easy to take charge of your weight and keep from packing on the menopause middle. Everything can go haywire during menopause when you overconsume high-glycemic carbohydrates and don't eat the correct food ratios for your changing body.

Once you achieve the proper food proportions, the next step is portion control. When you combine these two elements, you will start noticing your perfect weight emerge!

PORTION CONTROL

One of the hardest adjustments during the menopausal transition is changing the size of your food portions. For me, this was one of the most challenging lifestyle adjustments.

During the menopause transition, you must eat three small meals and two to three snacks every day, following the new food ratios (40% carbs, 35% protein, 25% fats) and using these portions:

CORRECT FOOD PORTIONS

Protein: Size and thickness of your palm—4–6 oz.

Carbs: Size of your fist (wrist to knuckles) or tennis ball—1 cup raw, ½ cup cooked or medium size

Fats: Size of your thumb

Water: 6–8 8-oz. glasses

Coffee: Less than 2 cups per day

Alcohol: Less than 6 oz. per day

MAKEOVER TIPS

- Fill over a third of your plate with lean protein, and the rest with low-glycemic carbohydrates, and sprinkle on some healthy fat.
- Purchase smaller plates. This strategy really helped me think I had a full plate of food.
- When preparing your weekly food plan, each meal should follow the Menopause Makeover Food Pyramid.

THE CALORIE COP: YOUR FRIENDLY PORTION-CONTROL ENFORCEMENT

During your Menopause Makeover, you should count your calories daily. This will require some effort, but the payoff is that you will see firsthand whether or not you are overeating. Even overeating healthy foods can add weight. This exercise will help you learn to adjust your portion sizes. After tracking your calories for a couple of weeks, you'll start to notice if your eating habits and portion sizes are working in your favor. I discovered two weeks into my makeover that I was overeating a favorite snack—veggies and hummus. Hummus is a wonderful snack, but it is high in calories.

We will discuss calories more in Chapter 10, and then calculate your calorie intake in Chapter 11. Then you will apply this information in your daily food portion of your 12-Week Essential Planner.

THE THERMIC EFFECT OF FOOD: YOUR SECRET WEAPON

When you follow the Menopause Makeover Food Pyramid, you will be using the thermic effect of food to help burn off that stubborn menopause belly fat. The thermic effect of food is the amount of energy it takes your body to digest food.

Thermic Effect for:

    Proteins: About 30%

    Carbohydrates: About 20%

    Fats: About 3%

Your body is using more energy to digest protein, helping you speed up your metabolism. A higher metabolism is your secret weapon to weight loss and good health. Knowing what foods speed up your metabolism can help you lose weight and burn that belly fat. We will calculate the thermic effect of food for your Menopause Makeover in Chapter 11.

SUPPLEMENTS

The best way to achieve nutritional health is by eating a diet rich in vitamins and minerals. Our bodies require more than 45 vitamins and minerals to maintain good health. Many of us do not consume a healthy diet, so there can be benefits to taking supplements. Supplements can have positive benefits during the menopausal transition. See Appendix B in the back of the book for a chart of dietary supplements.

Your body was designed to absorb nutrients from food sources. Consuming a healthy diet that includes natural food sources is the healthiest choice. Taking a daily multivitamin with minerals can be a good option as a supplement to a healthy diet. Discuss all supplement choices with your health-care provider. Vitamins and minerals can affect your health if combined with certain drugs; and many medications deplete your body of essential nutrients.

If you have health concerns, such as kidney stones, high cholesterol, high blood pressure or heart disease, notify your doctor of any new supplements added to your daily plan. If you are taking high dosages of aspirin daily, consult your doctor before adjusting your supplements.

Calcium with Vitamin D

During menopause it is advisable to take calcium and vitamin D for bone health. Calcium combined with vitamin D can help prevent osteoporosis.

Calcium plus vitamin D has been shown to reduce bone loss in healthy postmenopausal women, and also in postmenopausal women with substantial bone loss. All women should take 600 mg calcium and 400 IU vitamin D *twice* daily with food. The most common types of calcium supplements contain either calcium carbonate or calcium citrate. In general, both are adequately absorbed if taken with meals, but for some women calcium carbonate may cause constipation or gas. Taking calcium plus vitamin D daily is a good lifetime habit to form. Place your calcium/vitamin D in a pretty bowl and leave it out on the kitchen table, so you always remember to take your daily dose with a meal. Discuss calcium with vitamin D choices with your practitioner. There is more information on bone health in Chapter 4.

• • • MENOPAUSE MAKEOVER PLANNER ENTRY • • •

Record daily supplements in your
daily meal plan on page 363.

===

FEEDING THE NEW YOU

Making healthy food choices can change your life. Eating fast food and processed food, and overeating unhealthy foods, will only continue to contribute to a miserable menopause experience. Your food choices may be one of the most important changes you can make; healthy food choices will benefit you the rest of your life.

Once you start properly feeding the healthy girl hiding under a fat suit, your perfect weight will emerge. Many menopause symptoms may disappear, and your emotional health and self-esteem may improve, too. Eating the proper foods in the correct amounts will help you achieve a healthy weight.

Making smart decisions regarding food for your 12-Week Menopause Makeover is often the most difficult part of managing menopause. If you reach for food for emotional support, now is the time to challenge yourself and conquer those emotional issues. Remember, you can set yourself free with food!

KEEPING A DIARY AND CREATING A FOOD PLAN

Part of *The Menopause Makeover* plan is to keep a daily food diary and a weekly food plan. A daily food diary is a powerful tool for holding you accountable to your goals. Ladies who use a food diary lose almost twice the weight as those who do not. Your food diary will help identify areas that need improvement, so you can make necessary changes. Eating a healthy diet, maintaining a healthy weight and exercising may reduce your risk of disease.

There are food plan templates in Chapter 13, the Essential Planner. Design your food plans weekly. Having a plan is important, so you can achieve your food goals.

• • • MENOPAUSE MAKEOVER PLANNER ENTRY • • •

Make food and menu choices before your start each week. Prepare a shopping list that honors that plan using the sample list in the Essential Planner. Review a sample food plan on pages 350-353 of the Essential Planner.

Fill in the blank food plan on pages 354-355 with your weekly food choices, following your daily calorie intake.

MAKEOVER TIPS

- Eat the correct combination of foods (35% protein, 40% carbs, 25% fat) at every meal.
- Always eat within an hour of waking up.
- Eat 3 meals, and 2–3 snacks per day.
- Don't let yourself get hungry; never let more than 4 hours go by without eating.
- Drink lots of water.
- Have no more than one glass of alcohol per day.
- Have no more than 2 cups of coffee or other caffeinated drinks per day.
- Take your calcium and vitamin D twice daily.
- Get plenty of sleep.
- Record everything you eat and drink in your 12-Week Planner.
- Do not salt food or prepare food with salt.
- Enjoy healthy snacks with plenty of filling fiber.
- Watch your portions when eating out and avoid simple carbs like the bread basket. If the portion is too large, ask the waiter to take half and wrap it up for lunch the next day.
- Brown-bag a healthy lunch to stick to your food plan. You will save money and calories!
- If you are having a bad food day, don't beat yourself up; just get back on the plan the next day.
- Reward yourself when you have success. Go shopping for a pair of sexy shoes, rather than treating yourself to ice cream.

MAKEOVER TAKE-ACTION LIST

- Clear the kitchen of any foods not on your list of good proteins, carbohydrates and fats.
- Go to the grocery store with your shopping list of healthy foods, and purchase only foods listed on your food plan.
- If you're cooking for your family, start preparing meals following your plan. Making healthy food choices is good for the whole family.
- Start incorporating ways to cope with stress daily.
- If you are an emotional eater, identify your emotional triggers and confront them.
- Be honest when answering why you may be hiding under a fat suit. Discuss this with a close friend. Getting outside input may help you answer this question.

IN YOUR ESSENTIAL PLANNER

- Record nutritional goals on page 309.
- Select your preferred healthy protein, fat, carbohydrate and fiber choices and add them to your shopping list on page 357.
- Tape a copy of the Menopause Makeover Food Pyramid to your refrigerator door.
- Record all food intake daily in your 12-Week Planner on page 364.
- Prepare food plans each week, using the sample on page 354.
- Track your nutritional-goals progress daily in your 12-Week Planner.

chapter 4

Step Three: Exercise It Off:
You Think Hot Flashes Are Bad?
Now It's Time to Burn, Baby, Burn!

I created my own version of the seven dwarfs to describe my menopausal body: saggy, droopy, baggy, lumpy, frumpy, flabby and hefty! It wasn't enough to just eat healthfully, I wanted to look and feel healthy, and that meant adding exercise to my lifestyle.

Waking up at the crack of dawn and stuffing myself into an out-of-date, neon-colored exercise outfit, I'd dash out of the house, hiding under a big floppy hat, to begin power walking. Once I made a promise to feed and exercise my healthy self, I decided that power walking would be the only exercise I had the strength to actually endure. After months of pigging out and feeling sorry for myself, I had lost my endurance, lung capacity and muscle tone. Not to mention that my joints were not accustomed to carrying around my extra weight. I was embarrassed about my body. There was no way I was going to a gym or yoga class with walls of mirrors where others could witness my mushy, lumpy body trying to hide under a muumuu T-shirt.

With a spring in my power walking step, assuming my commitment and good attitude were all it was going to take to get healthy again, I was huffing and puffing after just 15 minutes at a slow pace. My heart was pounding, and I was drenched in sweat.

My health was in serious jeopardy. How was I ever going to get my strength back? It took two weeks, five days a week, to finally power walk 15 minutes without feeling doomed. I thought exercise was supposed to feel invigorating. Yet all I felt was discouraged.

After building some endurance, I increased the time I power walked and increased my pace, as well as my intensity, every day until I started seeing results. The endorphins were flowing again, and I felt happier. I could feel my strength coming back. Each week my fat suit slowly unzipped. There were days I dragged myself out of the house, dreading the workout. It was hard work. It took more than great effort. It took getting educated. I needed to understand my body and why it was failing me during menopause. I thought hot flashes were bad, but exercise was an uphill battle! After three months of exercise, I slipped back into my skinny jeans. Adding exercise to your daily schedule can increase the number of years you will live, it feels good and it helps you look good.

We live in a society that supports and promotes youth. Youthful, firm bodies are used to sell shampoo, clothes, cars and beauty products. We hardly ever see a real-looking 50-year-old woman in a shampoo ad. Even the "older" models are likely to have unnaturally skinny bodies. It is discouraging to be slapped in the face with billboards, magazine ads, commercials, TV shows and movies starring the young and the beautiful. It can make it twice as difficult to think there is hope of getting back into shape, reclaiming your health and beauty.

The good news is that once you add exercise to your daily routine, you have taken an enormous step for your health. A regular exercise routine will help you fight the clock and will relieve a number of menopause symptoms, including depression, crankiness, joint aches, muscle tension, high blood pressure, fatigue and anxiety as well as age-related concerns.

This chapter will cover exercise information needed to make choices for your personal Menopause Makeover. You will have the tools necessary to design an exercise plan that fits into your lifestyle. If you want to feel good, look good, conquer many diseases and age more gracefully, you must incorporate daily exercise. Without exercise, the quality of your survival declines and menopausal symptoms can increase. Who wants to be a menopausal blob of flab, inviting age and disease?

EXERCISE: YOUR FOUNTAIN OF YOUTH

Not only can daily exercise lower blood pressure and cholesterol, help you lose weight, slow or prevent osteoporosis and reduce anxiety, but *not* exercising actually increases your risk of many preventable diseases, including heart disease, certain cancers and type 2 diabetes.

Studies confirm that 20 to 30 minutes of exercise a day not only helps you live longer, but healthier. During exercise you breathe more deeply, increasing the amount of oxygen in your bloodstream; your heart beats harder, increasing the blood flow to your lungs and muscles, and helping carry away waste products; and your body releases endorphins, the feel-good hormones. You can't get enough endorphins during menopause!

Tragically, knowing the benefits of exercise is not enough—you have to actually go out and do it. Most of us do not have the time or the desire to include exercise in our daily routine, but the benefits are worth the effort. As we age—losing muscle mass and a youthful metabolism—menopause throws in a whole new set of challenges. During "the change" it may seem as if every day a new physical ailment crops up—night sweats, muscle aches or moodiness. Exercise can help with all of this.

If you are a baby boomer determined not to look mortality in the face, then exercise can be your fountain of youth.

BENEFITS OF EXERCISE

Lowers blood pressure	Strengthens your lungs
Increases bone density	Increases your stamina
Increases strength	Reduces anxiety and stress
Regulates blood sugar	Improves self-esteem
Strengthens your heart	Increases your metabolism

Improves digestive function	Strengthens your joints and ligaments
Increases good cholesterol and decreases bad cholesterol	Strengthens your immune system
Can enhance sexual pleasure	Lowers the risk of some cancers
Lowers risk of type 2 diabetes	Lowers the risk of heart disease
Increases general mobility	Builds healthy muscles, bones and joints
Burns calories	
Helps you feel healthier and happier	

HEART HEALTH

One of the greatest benefits of exercise is having a healthy heart. The leading killer of American women is heart attack. More than five times as many women die of heart attacks than from breast cancer. Menopause is associated with an increased risk of heart disease, making exercise that much more important.

What does menopause have to do with heart health?

After menopause, your risk of cardiovascular disease and high blood pressure significantly increases. At this time, there is still controversy, suggesting estrogen may provide cardioprotective benefits of estrogen. Throw in factors such as aging, a family history of heart disease, smoking, excessive alcohol consumption, a poor diet with too much salt intake, obesity and stress, and your risk of suffering from heart disease and high blood pressure increases.

What is blood pressure?

Over 39 million women have high blood pressure. Blood pressure is the force of blood against your artery walls. When you heart pumps blood out, it is called *systolic* pressure. When your heart is at rest between the beats, it is called *diastolic* pressure. When your doctor takes a blood pressure reading, the top, or first number is the systolic pressure, and the bottom, or second, number is the diastolic pressure. Normal blood pressure is equal to or less than 120/80.

High blood pressure is known as the silent killer because there are no symptoms and yet it can increase your risk of stroke, heart failure, kidney failure or heart attack. Age and genetics are the most common causes of high blood pressure. Weight gain and fluid retention can also be contributing factors.

There's good news, though: exercise can lower your blood pressure. If you suffer from high blood pressure, add exercise to your daily routine, even if you are on blood pressure medication. Lifestyle changes may delay or reduce your risk of heart disease and high blood pressure. Regular exercise will build a stronger heart, pumping more blood with less effort, and that means less pressure on your arteries. Committing to daily exercise may help you avoid blood pressure medications altogether. Monitor your blood pressure daily and discuss strategies to manage high blood pressure with your doctor.

Start exercising your body...
Your heart will love you for it!

BONE HEALTH

Weight-bearing and resistance exercises are the only exercises that can actually enhance bone growth and stop bone loss. When you do weight-bearing or resistance exercises, you force your muscles to work against gravity. The exercise causes your muscles to contract against the bone. Bone is living tissue, and this contraction stimulates new bone growth, so your bones actually grow stronger and denser.

Weight-bearing and resistance exercises also make it possible for bones to absorb more calcium. After the age of 30, women begin to lose bone mass and the risk of osteoporosis increases with menopause. Do not be a victim of poor bone health. Most of us want a tight butt and a firm tummy; but without strong bones, both are impossible. You need healthy bones to carry your body around the rest of your life. There is no cure for osteoporosis, but it is treatable. Make a commitment to your bone health and exercise!

Weight-bearing Exercises		Resistance/Strengthening Exercises	
Jogging	Tennis	Weightlifting	Weight machines
Step aerobics	Climbing stairs	Elastic tubing	
Dancing	Hiking	Push-ups	Free weights
Power walking	Jumping		

If you have osteoporosis

If you have a diagnosis of osteoporosis, consult with your health-care provider before starting a new exercise program. Your doctor might recommend low-impact exercises, like walking or swimming laps, and may also advise you against exercise that involves twisting, reaching or bending the spine.

INCREASED METABOLISM

One of the greatest benefits of exercise is that it can increase your metabolism. Your muscles burn 10 to 12 calories per pound, per 24-hour period, even while you are sleeping. During menopause, you lose muscle mass, so on top of weight gain, your metabolism slows.

The good news is that muscle burns more calories than fat, and increases your metabolism. Now is the time to start toning your muscles so you can raise your metabolism.

Focus on being healthy.

THE MENOPAUSE MAKEOVER EXERCISE FORMULA

Now you know the great things exercise can do for your body. So how do you get started? First you need to understand the different types of exercises you can do.

THREE TYPES OF EXERCISE

There are three ways to exercise:

1. *Flexibility exercises* reduce the risk of exercise-related injuries and maintain joint range of motion, so you can enjoy both cardiovascular and strength-training activities.

2. *Strength training* using weight-bearing or resistance exercises, can strengthen muscles, burning fat, increasing lean muscle mass, boosting metabolism and strengthening bones.

3. *Cardiovascular exercise* at your target heart rate can speed up metabolism and burn calories.

Five to six days a week you will do 5 minutes to 10 minutes of stretching to maintain flexibility. Then you will add twenty to thirty minutes of cardio, at your target heart rate (see page 127) for endurance and overall health. Two to three times a week, add strength training to build muscle tone. All you have to do is exercise 40 minutes most days of the week. That equals one TV show, the time to pack the kids' lunches (teach them how to make lunch), time to pick up the house in the morning (ask your partner to help, so you can exercise), or time on the phone with a friend (chat while you are power walking). Making time for exercise is possible. Consider exercise a Menopause Makeover prescription!

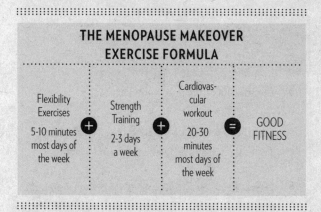

THE MENOPAUSE MAKEOVER EXERCISE FORMULA

Flexibility Exercises

5-10 minutes most days of the week

+

Strength Training

2-3 days a week

+

Cardiovascular workout

20-30 minutes most days of the week

=

GOOD FITNESS

FLEXIBILITY EXERCISES

Many of us rush into exercise routines without making time for proper stretching. Flexible muscles can reduce the chances of injury. As we age, our tendons and ligaments begin to stiffen, limiting our range of motion and making it painful to move. Stretching can stimulate the production of lubricants between the connective tissue fibers, reversing some of these effects of aging.

Always warm up a few minutes before stretching. You can turn the heat up, take a hot shower, walk around, march in place—just don't start stretching with tense muscles. Get your blood moving first allowing you to do your stretching routine with reduced risk of injury. Warm muscles are more pliable than cold ones.

MAKEOVER TIPS

- Stretch slowly.
- Commit yourself to proper technique.
- Breathe out at the maximum part of stretch.
- Do not bounce.
- Breathe naturally, do not hold your breath.
- Try to stretch a little farther on each stretch, during the exhale.
- Hold a stretch 10–15 seconds if you are a beginner, and work your way up to 30 seconds per stretch as your muscles become more flexible.

WHEN YOU FIRST START, GO SLOWLY, FOCUSING ON PROPER TECHNIQUE.

Benefits of stretching

- Reduces muscle tension.
- Increases body coordination.
- Keeps muscles supple.
- Does not cause pain when done correctly.
- Warms up muscles.
- Can reduce stress, feels relaxing.
- Feels good.
- Reduces risk of exercise-related injuries.
- Easy to learn.
- Maintains range of motion.
- Can be done anywhere and any time.
- Can prevent other injuries.
- Enhances flexibility.
- Enhances overall body image.
- Increases body temperature and heart rate.
- Develops body awareness.
- Increases ability to achieve physical relaxation.

STRENGTH TRAINING

The best way to strengthen muscles is to add resistance. When you fatigue a muscle or muscle group, lactic acids build up, causing a burning sensation. This is a wake-up call to those unused muscles to start working again. Your body will begin to synthesize new tissue to meet the demands you are putting on that muscle. Toning up a muscle requires progressive muscle resistance. Introducing more weight than the muscle can handle will help it grow stronger. Unlike cardio, where you work your body for a longer period, strength training puts stress on the muscle for a shorter period but at a higher intensity. Aging during the menopause transition results in loss of lean muscle mass; strength training will restore your muscle tissue. Toning those flabby arms, jiggly belly and wiggly booty will not only give you added strength, but your self-esteem will skyrocket, too!

Benefits of strength training

- Builds muscle.
- Burns calories, raises metabolism.
- Increases endurance and strength.
- Promotes bone health.
- Improves flexibility and coordination.
- Improves self-esteem.

Once you add strength training to your exercise routine you will witness how quickly your body adapts: You'll see changes before you know it.

Common strength equipment: weight machines (gym or home-gym models), free weights (dumbbells and barbells), resistance bands (elastic tubing with handles and elastic bands), or using your body weight (pull-ups and push-ups).

MAJOR MUSCLE GROUPS	
UPPER BODY	**LOWER BODY**
Chest: Pectorals, known as pecs	**Outer thighs:** Hip abductors
Shoulders: Deltoids, known as delts, rotator cuff	**Inner thighs:** Leg adductors
Back: Trapezius and latissimus dorsi, known as traps and lats	**Buttocks:** Gluteus maximus, known as glutes
Lower back: Erector spinae	**Quadriceps:** Known as quads

Arms: Biceps, triceps, forearms	**Hamstrings:** Known as hams
Abdominals: Rectus abdominis, known as abs	**Shins:** Tibialis anterior
Obliques and waist: Internal and external obliques	**Calves:** Gastrocnemius and soleus

Exercise the larger muscles first, so you do not exhaust the smaller muscle groups that are needed to exercise the larger muscles. Rest a day between each group.

Creating a strength-training routine

An easy way to organize your strength training routine is to divide the upper and lower body (abs included in the lower-body routine) and work them every other day.

SAMPLE STRENGTH TRAINING ROUTINE	
MONDAY	Upper body (back, chest, shoulders, triceps, biceps)
TUESDAY	Rest
WEDNESDAY	Lower body (glutes, quads, hams, calves, abs)
THURSDAY	Rest
FRIDAY	Upper body (back, chest, shoulders, triceps, biceps)
SATURDAY	Rest
SUNDAY	Rest

Creating a strength-training formula

Now all you need to do is put it all together into a series of reps and sets. A *rep* is a repetition of the same resistance exercise. A *set* is the chosen number of repetitions of that resistance exercise in a row. Rest 30 to 90 seconds between each set. If you are a beginner, start with a 90 second rest between sets.

MAKEOVER TIPS

- Don't hold your breath.
- Hold dumbbell by the center of the handle, except for the overhead extensions.
- Choose weights that are heavy enough to get through the scheduled number of reps. If the weight is not heavy enough, you will not stress the muscle enough to rebuild it.
- Rest 30–90 seconds between sets.
- Breathe in through your nose and out through your mouth. Breathe with full inhalations and exhalations. Exhale when your muscles are tightening.
- If you want to make this a cardio workout while strength training, do not rest between sets.
- Wear comfy clothes that breathe—not too baggy and not too tight.

COMMON STRENGTH-TRAINING FORMULAS

Beginner	Intermediate	Advanced
1 set 10 reps	2–3 sets 10–12 reps	3 sets 12–15 reps

For your abs, do 10 to 25 reps at your appropriate "set" level

When your workout becomes easy, add weight and change your routine to keep it interesting and to stimulate the muscles.

CARDIOVASCULAR EXERCISE

Once you select an enjoyable cardio activity that fits into your lifestyle, make a commitment to do it most days a week.

Benefits of cardiovascular activity

- Relieves stress.
- Improves heart function.
- Reduces the risk of heart disease.
- Improves blood cholesterol and triglyceride levels.
- Reduces the risk of osteoporosis.
- Improves muscle tone.
- Increases production of endorphins.
- Reduces the risk of diabetes.
- Helps with weight management.
- Increases lung capacity.
- Helps you sleep better.
- Boosts mood.

MAKEOVER TIPS

- Discuss your program with your doctor.
- Schedule cardio workouts on your calendar.
- Aim to do at least 20–30 continuous minutes most days of the week.
- Make sure you are using good gear or equipment.

TOP 10 CARDIO EXERCISES
Calories burned in 30 minutes, for a 145-pound woman

Exercise	Calories	Exercise	Calories
Step Aerobics	400 calories	Cross-country skiing	330 calories
Bicycling	200 – 500 calories	Running	300 calories
Swimming	400 calories	Elliptical machine	300 calories
Playing racquetball	400 calories	Rowing	300 calories
Rock climbing	380 calories	Walking	180 calories

If you are jogging or power walking, owning a good pair of shoes is important to avoid injury. Also, consider incorporating music, reading or watching TV during your training, so you don't get bored. Wrangle a friend and have fun chatting during your session. Don't forget to mix it up. If you are working out at the gym, switch between the elliptical cross-trainer and the treadmill. If you power walk in your neighborhood, try hiking or biking with a friend for variety.

SAMPLE WORKOUT SCHEDULE	
MONDAY	Warm-up/stretch, strength training, cardio
TUESDAY	Warm-up/stretch, cardio
WEDNESDAY	Warm-up/stretch, strength training, cardio
THURSDAY	Warm-up/stretch, cardio
FRIDAY	Warm-up/stretch, strength training, cardio
SATURDAY	Warm-up/stretch, cardio
SUNDAY	Rest

WHEN TO EXERCISE AND FOR HOW LONG

You can exercise any time of the day. Many people prefer to do it first thing in the morning, and start the day fresh. Others like to exercise at the end of their day to release tension. And others split up their exercise routines between morning and evening to work it into their busy schedules. The days you incorporate strength training, I recommend two sessions if you need to break up your routine. Do your stretches and strength training in the morning, and 20 to 30 minutes of cardio later in the day, or vice versa. If you plan to do this, remember to warm up a few minutes before your cardio segment.

Do not eat a heavy meal just before exercising. Consume something light, like an apple for energy, before your exercise routine. Eat a balanced meal within two hours of completing your exercise regimen.

BURNING CALORIES

Every time I clean and vacuum the house, I feel good knowing that my house looks great, and I just zapped a couple hundred calories. That equals a glass of red wine or a small yummy dessert. See where your brain can go when you have the information? You may ask, "If it is all about calories, why don't I just decrease my food intake and who needs exercise?" Do you cut food calories? Or increase exercise?

The *Journal of Clinical Endocrinology and Metabolism* and the USDA confirm that weight loss is about the calories. The more you burn, baby, burn, the more weight you'll lose. In fact, consuming 500 fewer calories per day (just add a power walk and cut out a bagel) and you will lose a pound a week. I have found it easier to negotiate my day knowing I can use both food and exercise calories to meet my goals. Plus, exercise tones your muscles, and increases your heart and breathing rates, translating into good health and healthy self-esteem. Cutting only food calories can be challenging, but exercise and physical activity are wonderful tools to burn extra calories.

This lifestyle change is about balance, making a daily commitment to your health. Have a plan every day. Think about what you will be eating and when you'll get your workout in. If you have time, squeeze in a fun physical activity, like a walk during lunch. Even if you don't want to lose weight, exercise will help you maintain a healthy weight and lifestyle.

I discovered early in my quest for good health during menopause that not all women burn the same number of calories per activity. It depends on your weight and the intensity level you are moving at.

Do not compare yourself, or your exercise results, with anyone else. Your goals and your results are unique to you.

CALORIES BURNED PER HOUR
> CIRCLE 3 ACTIVITIES THAT YOU CAN DO FOR YOUR MENOPAUSE MAKEOVER

SELECT YOUR WEIGHT CATEGORY	130 LB	155 LB	190 LB
Aerobics, general	354	422	518
Bicycling, less than 10mph, leisure	236	281	345
Bicycling, stationary—moderate effort	413	493	604
Bowling	177	211	259
Canoeing, rowing—moderate effort	413	493	604
Cleaning house—general	207	246	302
Dancing—general	266	317	388
Exercise equipment, cardio	354	422	518
Gardening	295	352	431
Golfing, general	236	281	345

CALORIES BURNED PER HOUR

SELECT YOUR WEIGHT CATEGORY	130 LB	155 LB	190 LB
Health club excercise—general	325	387	474
Hiking, cross-country	354	422	518
Horse grooming	354	422	518
Horse riding—general	236	281	345
Horse riding—trotting	382	457	561
Jogging—general	413	493	604
Kayaking	295	352	431
Rope jumping—moderate	590	704	863
Rowing, stationary—moderate effort	413	493	604
Running, 5 mph (12-min. mile)	472	563	690
Running, 5.2 mph (11.5-min. mile)	531	633	776
Running, 6 mph (10-min. mile)	590	704	863
Running, 6.7 mph (9-min. mile)	648	774	949
Running—general	472	563	690
Running—in place	472	563	690
Running upstairs	885	1056	1294

CALORIES BURNED PER HOUR

SELECT YOUR WEIGHT CATEGORY	130 LB	155 LB	190 LB
Sailing, boat/board, windsurfing—general	177	211	259
Skating, ice—general	413	493	604
Skating, roller	413	493	604
Skiing, cross-country—moderate effort	472	563	690
Skiing, snow—general	413	493	604
Snowshoeing	472	563	690
Softball or baseball, fast or slow pitch	295	352	431
Stretching, hatha yoga	236	281	345
Surfing, body or board	177	211	259
Swimming laps, freestyle—light/moderate effort	472	563	690
Swimming, leisurely—general	354	422	518
Swimming, treading water—moderate effort	236	281	345
Table tennis	236	281	345
Tai chi	236	281	345
Teaching aerobics class	354	422	518
Tennis—doubles	354	422	518

CALORIES BURNED PER HOUR

SELECT YOUR WEIGHT CATEGORY	130 LB	155 LB	190 LB
Tennis—general	413	493	604
Tennis—singles	472	563	690
Volleyball—beach	472	563	690
Walking, 2.0 mph—slow pace	148	176	216
Walking, 3.0 mph—moderate pace, walking dog	207	246	302
Walking, 3.5 mph—uphill	354	422	518
Walking, 4.0 mph—very brisk pace	236	281	345
Walking—grass track	295	352	431
Walking—upstairs	472	563	690
Water aerobics, water calisthenics	236	281	345
Waterskiing	354	422	518
Water volleyball	177	211	259
Weight lifting or body building—vigorous effort	354	422	518
Weight lifting—light or moderate effort	177	211	259

Source: Department of Health and Family Services, State of Wisconsin. Calories Burned Per Hour. 2005. Available at: http://dhs.wisconsin.gov/health/physicalactivity/pdf_files/Caloriesperhour.pdf.

The good news is that you burn calories all day during normal activities, too. But don't think this is an excuse to skip the gym!

DAILY ACTIVITIES WITH CALORIES BURNED PER HOUR

Sleeping	55	Knitting	85	Driving	110
Eating	85	Sitting	85	Office Work	140
Sewing	85	Standing	100	Housework	150

FINDING YOUR TARGET HEART RATE

How do you know if you are working hard enough to reap the benefits? One of the easiest ways to check your intensity is to monitor your heart rate. The target heart rate (THR) is your pulse rate per minute. When you train within your THR, you strengthen the cardiovascular system by exercising the heart, and increasing blood and oxygen flow to your tissues. Your target heart rate is calculated at 60 to 80 percent of your maximum heart rate (MHR).

If you are a beginner, calculate the formula at 60 percent. When your routine becomes easy for you, then move up to 70 percent, then 80 percent, as you get stronger.

If you are not using a cardio exercise machine with a heartrate monitor, you can purchase a heart rate monitor from $25 to $350. You can also take your pulse during exercising. Lightly place your two middle fingers on your throat at the jugular vein or on your wrist over your pulse. Count your heartbeat for six seconds, and add a zero to that number.

The "talk test" is another good way to determine the intensity of your workout. If you can talk but are a little winded, then you are in your target zone. If you are completely winded and can barely talk, slow down. If chatting is too easy, step it up a notch (the cardio, not the chatting, that is). Always discuss your exercise choices with your doctor.

AVOIDING INJURIES

I was excited about starting a new exercise routine for my Menopause Makeover, so I jumped in with full effort, thinking my body was still 20 years old. In the first yoga class I took, I injured my rotator cuff (shoulder injury) doing Down Dog pose with too much energy for too long without the strength to support it. I visited the doctor, he injected cortisone, it healed, and then I went back to yoga class, only to injure my lumbar 4/5 discs on a spinal twist.

Why was I getting injuries all of a sudden? First, with aging, ligaments and tendons are not as pliable. Second, my brain was acting like it was a 20-year-old not a 50-year-old. When you start the 12-Week Menopause Makeover Exercise Plan, start out slow and easy. Better to prevent an injury from the start. If you have a history

HOW TO CALCULATE YOUR TARGET HEART-RATE ZONE

{ Step #1 }

Calculate your Maximum Heart Rate
(upper limit of what your heart can handle during your workout)

---

220 – your age = **MHR**

> Example for a 49-year-old woman: 220 – 49 = 171 MHR

{ Step #2 }

Calculate your Target Heart Rate

MHR x .60 = **THR**
(low-end range)

MHR x .70 = **THR**
(middle range)

MHR x .80 = **THR**
(high range)

> **EXAMPLE** for a 49-year-old woman:

Her low-end range (60%)	171 (MHR) x .60 = 102.6
Her middle range (70%)	171 (MHR) x .70 = 119.7
Her high range (80%)	171 (MHR) x .80 = 136.8

This 49-year-old's target heart rate is between
102.6 and 136.8 beats per minute.

with an injury, such as knee or back issues, respect your injury. Do not overdo it. Speak to your health-care practitioner before starting a new exercise plan. Whether you suffer from a torn ligament, muscle strain or joint concerns, make sure your daily exercise does not strain an existing injury. Always allow your injury to heal before putting stress on it again through exercise. You do not want an injury to turn into a permanent health concern.

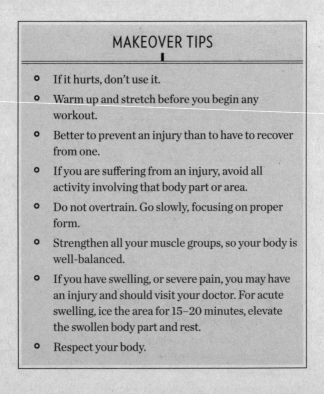

MAKEOVER TIPS

- If it hurts, don't use it.
- Warm up and stretch before you begin any workout.
- Better to prevent an injury than to have to recover from one.
- If you are suffering from an injury, avoid all activity involving that body part or area.
- Do not overtrain. Go slowly, focusing on proper form.
- Strengthen all your muscle groups, so your body is well-balanced.
- If you have swelling, or severe pain, you may have an injury and should visit your doctor. For acute swelling, ice the area for 15–20 minutes, elevate the swollen body part and rest.
- Respect your body.

CHECK YOUR POSTURE

You can look pounds thinner and more confident with good posture. When you exercise, practice good posture. You know you have good posture when you can draw a straight line from your ear through your shoulder, hip and knee.

Sucking in your tummy and tucking in your tush on a regular basis will help strengthen your muscles and improve your appearance and mood. Whenever you walk, stand, sit and lie down, practice good posture. Once you begin your regular workout routine, having good posture will become automatic. Good posture will help prevent injuries during exercise, and you can look thinner and feel more confident.

STAYING MOTIVATED AND SETTING GOALS

One of the hardest commitments to make during your menopause transition is incorporating exercise into your daily routine. It is so much easier to sit on the couch and watch a movie, enjoying a pint of ice cream. Trust me: You will feel better adding exercise to your life. Your self-esteem will improve, your clothes will fit better, you will have added strength and you will add years to your life.

1. Choose 5 activities you like that you can incorporate into your lifestyle—anything from dancing, to power walking with the girls, to walking the dog, stair climbing or window cleaning.

2. Set realistic goals.

3. Record all physical activity in your 12-Week Menopause Makeover Planner.

4. Mix it up! This ensures that your body does not get used to the same activity and you no longer reap the benefits. Avoid boredom at all costs.

5. Schedule exercise in your 12-Week Menopause Makeover Planner.

6. If you are a procrastinator, and need motivation to get moving, attend scheduled classes.

7. Exercise at the same time every day, so it becomes part of your daily lifestyle.

8. Buy a cute exercise outfit, so you feel great working out.

9. Put together a music playlist on your iPod with upbeat tunes. Motivating music goes a long way toward keeping you on track.

10. Watch your favorite TV shows while working out at the gym or on your home machine.

11. If you only have 15–20 minutes, use the time for strength training or a cardio session. Twenty minutes is better than no activity.

12. If you work out at home, create a space you like and devote it to exercising.

13. Get an exercise buddy; socialize and burn calories together.

14. Exercise for a charity. Raise money for breast cancer; start training for Avon™'s 39-mile, 2-day

benefit to raise money for breast cancer research. A good cause is a great motivator!

15. Reward yourself when you see results. Enjoy a day of shopping or pamper yourself with a spa day.

> If your schedule is too busy for exercise, wake up half an hour earlier.

FIND THE RIGHT EXERCISE FOR YOU

If you are a person who needs a coach or leader, has energy in the afternoon, likes being social, prefers being indoors and isn't competitive, then joining a gym or taking a class (yoga, dancing) may be a good way to incorporate exercise into your lifestyle. Or get a group of friends together and alternate homes for a neighborhood power walk, and do your stretching and strength training together.

If you like the outdoors, do not need leadership, feel energized in the morning and prefer having some alone time, then you may benefit from a morning power walk or hike, combined with your stretching and strength training.

Honor yourself. Incorporating exercise into your lifestyle is a big commitment. You will need all odds in your favor.

QUIZ | What type of exercise person are you?

Would you prefer to have a coach tell you what to do, or do you like to be your own boss?

What time of day do you feel most energized? Morning? Afternoon? Evening?

Do you like to exercise with friends or solo?

Could you set up an area in your home to exercise? Or do you prefer to go to a gym or classroom?

Do you need a cheerleader to encourage you? Or can you motivate yourself?

Are you competitive with others in a class situation?

Do you like to exercise? If not, find a support team and organized exercise activities.

Would you prefer to get exercise through other activities, like dancing or hiking?

Are you an indoor or an outdoor person?

If you make a commitment to yourself, will you
honor it?

HOW HEALTHY ARE YOU?

One of the best ways to motivate yourself is to set goals
for improvement. Walking is a wonderful gauge to test
your overall aerobic health. Take this test and find out
how healthy you are. You can take this quiz using a
treadmill with computerized distance and time set-
tings, or mark off the distance in your neighborhood
by driving (note the odometer reading at each mile) and
time it yourself when walking.

> When exercising becomes a drag,
> ask a buddy to join you.

ONE-MILE WALK FITNESS TEST

Record how long it takes you to walk one mile, then use these guidelines to rate your fitness level:

Fitness Level	Time
Fantastic	less than 11:44
Really great	11:45-13:11
Above average	13:12-14:34
Average	14:35-16:04
Not so good	16:05-17:29
Poor	more than 17:30

A brisk walk, 3.5 to 4.5 miles an hour, has cardiovascular benefits. After you determine your quiz results, you will be able to set goals to improve your health through exercise. When I launched a daily exercise routine, I was walking a 17:45-minute mile—a poor health grade! Six months later, I was walking a 14-minute mile. Just do it, your body will thank you. Now I power through a 13-minute mile with ease. My new goal is the 11:30-minute mile.

CREATE YOUR OWN HOME GYM

Having exercise equipment at home can increase your odds of incorporating exercise into your lifestyle. Find an area in your home designated for your workouts.

I made a workout area in front of my bedroom mirror. I keep my exercise mat, dumbbells and chair next to the mirror. This equipment can be used for stretching, weight lifting with dumbbells and cardiovascular routines. The exercise enthusiast may choose to purchase a home gym and cardiovascular machine (treadmill, elliptical).

MENOPAUSE MAKEOVER HOME GYM EQUIPMENT			
Full-length mirror	Pedometer	Heart-rate monitor	Chair
Dumbbells	Yoga/exercise mat	Appropriate shoes	Towels

CREATE A SUPPORT TEAM

Working out with friends is a wonderful way to socialize while reaping the benefits of exercise. Working out with a friend is a fun way to honor your commitment to exercise. Plus, having a gym buddy is great motivation to stick to your exercise routine.

NO MORE EXCUSES

Are you struggling or resisting the exercise challenge? "I don't have time" was my biggest reason to not exercise. Then I moved to a new city when I got married, and my explanation became "The gym is too far." Once I decided to power walk, because the gym was 20 minutes away, my new excuse became "It is not safe to walk at night." Most of us have some pretty good excuses for not including exercise in our lifestyle.

MAKEOVER TIPS

- Schedule workouts with friends in advance.
- Set goals with friends; enjoy a little competition with a tempting reward for success (that all can enjoy).
- Join a walking club.
- Take classes at your gym.
- Locate a nightclub that gives free dance classes and book that evening with a group of friends with similar dance interests.
- Combine exercise with other activities (create a dog-walking group, for instance).

What's your excuse not to exercise?
Make a check next to your favorite excuses—and next time you go to use one, don't!

CHECKLIST	
YOUR FAVORITE EXCUSES	✓
Find exercise boring	
Do not have time to exercise	
Lack motivation and time management skills	
No confidence in my body	
Fear of being injured	
Exercise is an inconvenience	
Lack of support or encouragement	
No exercise location	
Were you the kid people made fun of during gym class?	

What is the solution to your excuse not to exercise?

How can you create a positive remedy for your resistance to exercising?

Exercise can be fun and social. Focus on doing activities you enjoy, include friends and you have a formula for success.

EXERCISE THE NEW YOU

Maximizing your workout will not only improve your overall health, it will give you a head start on battling menopausal weight gain, depression and saggy muscles. Exercise can also help you deal with uncomfortable menopause symptoms, like hot flashes, anxiety, joint pain and sleep disturbances. Plus, it reduces your risk of heart disease and osteoporosis!

REMEMBER

What you think, you become

Having support is a powerful tool

Positive thinking goes a long way

Have one good laugh session a day

Reward yourself when you see progress

MAKEOVER TIPS

- Record your daily activity in your 12-Week Planner.

- Have a small snack 15–30 minutes before your workout (apple, yogurt, low-fat cottage cheese).

- Drink water during your exercise routine.

- Find small ways to burn calories during the day: Take the stairs instead of the elevator, park your car at the far side of the mall parking lot or stretch while you watch TV.

- Always plan your week in advance and schedule your workouts. If your schedule opens up, throw in some stretches, cardio or strengthening exercises.

- Do not overtrain—take it slow and easy, yet get a good workout.

- Variety is the spice of life—try new routines and activities, add friends, get a new playlist on your iPod.

- Challenge yourself with intensity levels, times and new activities.

MAKEOVER TAKE-ACTION LIST

- Prepare an area of your house to build your home gym, or join a local gym.
- Work out most days of the week.
- Always warm up a few minutes before any exercise to avoid injury.
- Practice good posture.
- Record all exercise goals on page 311.
- Record your target heart rate on page 312, and track it daily in your planner.
- If you have high blood pressure, or cholesterol issues, record your levels on page 340.

IN YOUR ESSENTIAL PLANNER

- Record your selected workout routine in your Month-at-a-Glance Planner.
- Record daily workouts in your 12-Week Planner.
- List your workout buddies on page 339.
- Track your exercise progress in your Weekly Progress report.

chapter 5

Step Four: Mirror, Mirror on the Wall, Is That Me?
Customizing Your Beauty Routine

I have stopped complaining about my blurry vision. For years, I looked in the mirror and saw someone in her early thirties. Of course, I wasn't wearing my reading glasses, so my out-of-focus vision was a blessing in disguise. After months of hearing me complain about my vision while I was applying makeup, a friend suggested that I purchase a 5X-magnifying mirror. This solution was disastrous! Seeing myself in focus was horrifying. I looked like my mother! No offense, Mom. When did I get fine lines around my eyes? And those frown lines were now permanent fixtures hanging from my sagging cheeks and jowls.

The ugly truth is that menopause was taking its toll on my skin. The skin on my face was changing drastically; the skin on my arms looked like wrinkled dessert crepes; the skin around my belly resembled a squashed donut; and the skin that supported my tush had recently deflated, leaving a droopy booty. And, as if aging skin weren't bad enough, one morning I woke up to find a long black hair on my forehead. "It must be from my makeup brush!" When I went to brush it off, it remained attached. The one-inch black hair had sprung up overnight. A tweeze job followed by a stiff cup of coffee was the only solution.

With aging skin, declining vision, stray hairs and a changing figure, feeling in control of your beauty may seem impossible. Having worked with 40-something celebrities and their beauty teams during my television career, I realized I had some beauty secrets that needed dusting off. Years ago, a makeup artist confessed to me that her celebrity had a beauty secret that kept her skin gorgeous: weekly exfoliation. Years later, a costume designer quietly mentioned that his star looked ten pounds thinner because he had lowered her belt line. One of my greatest beauty discoveries happened when I entered the dressing room of a huge celebrity as she was having her microphone discreetly wired under her outfit. As the female sound person had the celebrity's dress pulled up to tape wires underneath, I sighted this beautiful over-50 star's toning undergarment (yep, a full-body girdle) from her bra to her thighs. When she caught me staring at her girdled body, she smiled and said, "One day you'll need one, too!" And she was right!

After months of serious exercise, my tummy was still a bowl of Jell-O—it was smaller, but loose and flabby. I purchased a sexy body-slimming suit with a built-in bra (inspired by that very wise movie star), and voilà! My perky boobs and booty returned. If you are wondering who that movie star was, I will go to my grave with her name, but not her beauty secrets!

When you have a few beauty and styling tips in your arsenal, your 5X-magnifying mirror can be your friend. And don't be afraid to hang up the full-length mirror again!

This chapter is packed with simple beauty and style tips, from skin-care tips to monthly teeth whitening. You will enter beauty and style appointments in your Month-at-a-Glance Planner, so you can accomplish beauty goals during your Menopause Makeover.

HELP, I'M TURNING INTO MY MOTHER!

A few years ago, while on a water-skiing trip, I was bending over the outboard motor at the back of the power-boat tossing a water ski to a friend in the water. The boat driver called out, "Staness, toss out just one ski." As I turned to hear his command I could see a lumpy, flabby butt in his rearview mirror. I thought, "My mom is not on this boat, so whose butt is that? She has the same swimsuit as I do." To my horror, it was *my* butt. I was in my forties, and I thought my booty was still sexy. My butt was now *my mother's butt*. Was I aging like my mother? My mother was starting to appear in my life everywhere. I started dressing like her to hide my ever-growing midsection and droopy butt. I noticed sagging skin under my chin, and some facial peach fuzz, just like Mom!

WHY IS MY SKIN WRINKLING AND SAGGING?

Thanks to aging and fluctuating hormones, I was quickly becoming my mother. Fortunately, I have a beautiful mother, but nothing was going to stop the inevitable— age and menopause.

During menopause we really start seeing the effects of aging. Your skin is supported by collagen and elastin fibers, which is why your skin looked so soft and contoured to your face before menopause. Throw in the loss of collagen, elastin and hyaluronic acid that happens naturally as you age, and you have a formula for wrinkles and looser skin. Hormones can affect the skin's physiology, with almost 30 percent of the skin's collagen depleted in the first five years after menopause.

When I discovered that changing hormones were to blame for the acceleration of wrinkles and saggy skin, I ran to my doctor, hoping for a huge dose of estrogen. What I discovered is that the FDA has not approved estrogen therapy to treat aging skin. There is no hard science to prove that estrogen therapy can improve the appearance of your skin. I personally saw visible changes when I began hormone therapy. I know for a fact that hormone therapy alleviated my miserable symptoms; perhaps my *feeling* better had a positive effect on my complexion.

If you were a sun worshipper, a smoker, or had bad eating habits, this can deplete more moisture, causing deeper wrinkles. If you used birth control pills or are currently on hormone therapy, you may be battling brown spots. Many women find new wrinkles cropping up, such as deep lines from smiling or frowning. Combine these frustrations with your skin's natural process of exfoliation, called desquamation, in which old cells slough off to make way for the new, and you have a dull-looking complexion. As if that were not enough, you can thank gravity for all that sagging. Recently, a menopausal friend asked, "If I hang upside down in gravity boots for an hour a day, will it stop the sagging?" Sadly, the answer is "no." Maybe a lifetime in space is the only answer to zero gravity.

HOW WILL YOU AGE?

We can't stop the aging process—even those of you running to the plastic surgeon cannot escape. I went on a beauty quest that would *embrace* my age, not disguise it. If you begin good beauty habits today, you can actually slow down the effects of aging.

Wouldn't it be nice to wave a magic wand and turn aging skin into youthful radiance? You cannot stop aging. Sorry, ladies, it bummed me out, too. You can, however, manage aging. Embrace the experience by arming yourself with the magic of good beauty habits.

There are two types of aging—internal and external. Our genes cause internal aging. Internal aging begins in our twenties, but signs do not appear for decades. Dry skin, fine wrinkles, thin skin and loss of underlying fat are examples of internal aging. Although we cannot stop internal aging, thankfully we can at least slow down external aging. External aging adds to our naturally occurring internal aging. The sun, gravity, facial expressions, sleeping positions and smoking are all external factors that accelerate aging.

The 25 age-embracing tips below do not include dermabrasion, laser resurfacing, microdermabrasion or chemical peels—procedures that produce a new top layer of skin, removing brown spots and fine wrinkles. We can slow the aging process with good beauty habits. Applying these anti-aging tips can erase years from your face.

QUIZ | How Will You Age?
25 Anti-Aging Tips

CHECK OFF THE AGE-EMBRACING GUIDELINES YOU PRACTICE	✓
1 › Wear sunscreen daily. The sun is your biggest enemy. Apply sunscreen of SPF 15 or greater 20 minutes prior to going outside.	
2 › Cleanse and moisturize your skin twice daily.	
3 › Use a retinol night cream.	
4 › Be sure to moisturize the delicate skin around your eyes. Facial moisturizers or a moisturizing face cream will do the job.	
5 › Remove makeup every night before going to bed.	
6 › Exfoliate your face regularly.	

QUIZ

CHECK OFF THE AGE-EMBRACING GUIDELINES YOU PRACTICE	✔
7 > Enjoy weekly hydrating facial masks.	
8 > Use anti-aging and antioxidant products in your skin-care regimen.	
9 > Massage your skin. It is good for blood circulation, relaxes muscles and can relieve signs of tiredness.	
10 > If you smoke, STOP.	
11 > Take omega-3 supplements.	
12 > Limit alcohol consumption.	
13 > Wear sunglasses. Squinting from the sun will only accelerate the manifestation of those lines around your eyes.	
14 > Avoid suntanning. If you want a tanned look, use facial bronzers or sunless tanners for a healthy summer glow.	
15 > Avoid really hot showers and baths.	
16 > Use detergent-free soaps for your face and body.	
17 > Use 2% hydroquinone topical over-the-counter cream to lighten subtle skin discoloration.	
18 > Treat yourself to a professional facial, and discuss a skin-care regimen for your skin type.	

QUIZ

CHECK OFF THE AGE-EMBRACING GUIDELINES YOU PRACTICE	✔
19 > Practice relaxation techniques. Second to sun damage, stress can age your skin.	
20 > Always wear a hat in the sun.	
21 > Sleep on a satin pillowcase to avoid facial creases, and get enough sleep.	
22 > Drink plenty of water.	
23 > Eat a healthy diet, rich in antioxidants (citrus fruits, blueberries, strawberries, green tea, red vegetables, fresh salads). Avoid salt, sugar, caffeine and fatty foods. Eat fiber. Take your supplements. Eat fish 3–4 times a week.	
24 > Exercise most days of the week.	
25 > Maintain a healthy weight.	

THE RESULTS
How many tips did you check off?

25	You go, girl. You will probably knock off 15 years from your age with these terrific beauty habits. Keep up the good work.
20	Very impressive. Do people ask if your daughter is your sister? Kick it up a notch and join your sisters in the "25" group. Or stay where you are and your good habits will knock off 10 years.
15	A good start. Add a few more tips, and join the ladies who ranked above you. Or continue the same strategy and notice 5 years knocked off your age.
10	Nice try, but you won't see the results you may be looking for as the years pass. Try adding 5 tips monthly to your regimen for the next 2–3 months.
5	Oh, girlfriend… You either have great genes, or you look like your grandmother. There is hope. Start adding some of these tips to your daily life, and fast. Depending on external factors in your life, it is never too late to begin practicing better grooming habits.
0	What freedom not to worry about your skin. That could be a good thing. But one of these days, you'll wish you'd taken better care of your skin! Warning: Wake up and slap on some sunscreen and moisturizer.

Beauty is more than skin deep—
beauty radiates from a happy spirit
and healthy body!

SKIN-CARE SOLUTIONS THAT TURN BACK THE CLOCK

Many women visit their dermatologist or plastic surgeon to remedy new wrinkles and saggy skin. I have witnessed many friends go through uncomfortable injections for wrinkles, chemical peels and full face-lifts only to be disappointed with the results. Not only were many of these procedures expensive, they were painful and involved weeks or months of recovery time.

Daily moisturizing, weekly exfoliation and wearing sunscreen can actually help turn back the clock of age, soften deep wrinkles and prevent brown spots. Weekly exfoliation can renew a dull complexion instantly. Moisturizing can soften wrinkles. If you want faster results, consult a dermatologist—see the Getting Professional Help section on page 157. First, let's review nonsurgical options available to maintain a healthy radiant skin.

NO MATTER YOUR AGE

Each age group has new skin concerns to address with an updated skin regimen.

In your 30s: Fine lines around the eyes. Frown and smiling lines begin to appear. Sleeping lines take longer to disappear. Spider veins may appear. You may begin to notice puffy eyes in the morning. Keep skin hydrated, and start using SPF 15+ daily.

In your 40s: Facial expression lines become deeper. The bags under your eyes become more prominent; your skin becomes drier and more sensitive; your neck looks crepey; your pores increase in size; you experience an increase or decrease in facial hair; you begin to see age spots, spider veins, rosacea and saggy skin.

In your 50s: Skin loses its elasticity faster. Wrinkles and deep folds may develop. The skin becomes thinner and more fragile. You may develop "jowls" where the skin on the cheeks sags and hangs down either side of the chin. Sun damage is unforgiving now; brown spots increase, as well as deep lines in the cheeks and around the eyes and mouth. The eyelids may also have developed a crepey appearance.

In your 60s and beyond: You may develop dry, itchy skin. Age spots, wrinkles and expression lines are etched into the face. Skin texture is no longer moist or supple. Skin is fragile and care must be taken to not tear it.

YOUR NEW SKIN-CARE REGIMEN

The skin is made up of two layers: The outer layer is called the *epidermis* and the inner layer is called the *dermis.* The inner layer contains nerve endings, blood vessels, sweat glands and the collagen and elastin that support your skin. The epidermis produces melanin (a pigment that is naturally present to varying degrees), and is constantly producing new skin cells to replace the ever-flaking dead skin cells. The skin is our body's protection from the environment—it regulates body temperature, stores water and fat, and prevents the entry of bacteria. Our skin is an important organ, and it is the one organ everyone can see. We all want beautiful, healthy skin.

Even if you have already started to notice some wrinkles, you can soften them with a new skin-care regimen. Beauty tips that worked before your menopausal transition will need to be updated. Intensive moisturizing, using anti-aging products with retinoid and antioxidant ingredients, consumption of water, exercise and a healthy diet can bring back your youthful luster inside and out.

During menopause you may experience dry, itchy skin as well as loss of skin elasticity. Beautiful skin begins with a good, daily skin-care regimen. Turn back the clock and reclaim your youthful skin with the correct skin-care regimen.

MENOPAUSE MAKEOVER SKIN REGIMEN

SKIN TYPE				
NORMAL	OILY	DRY	SENSITIVE	DEHYDRATED
CLEANSER				
Gentle cleansing gel or milk applied morning and night	Gentle cleansing gel or milk used for normal skin applied morning and night	Cleanser, lotion or cream for dry skin. Must be gently applied morning and night	Gentle milk or cream cleanser, applied morning and night	Gentle milk or gel cleanser applied morning and night
TONER				
Alcohol-free toner applied morning and night	Alcohol-free toner applied morning and night	Gentle alcohol-free toner applied morning and night	Mild toner for sensitive skin, applied morning and night	Hydrating toner applied morning and night

MENOPAUSE MAKEOVER SKIN REGIMEN

SKIN TYPE

NORMAL	OILY	DRY	SENSITIVE	DEHYDRATED
DAY CREAM				
Start using a daily moisturizer with SPF 15+ applied daily	Light, water-based moisturizer with SPF 15+ applied daily	Rich, oil-based moisturizer with SPF 15+ applied daily	Gentle daily moisturizer with SPF 15+ applied daily	Hydrating water-based moisturizer with SPF 15+ applied daily
NIGHT CREAM				
Light, nourishing night cream applied nightly	Use same daily moisturizer without sunscreen applied nightly	Oil-based moisturizer for night repair applied nightly	Wear your day cream at night, applied nightly	Deep-moisturizing night skin-care cream, to restore moisture loss, applied nightly
EXFOLIATE				
Use an exfoliating scrub or glycolic at 2% applied 1–2 times weekly	Use an exfoliating scrub applied 2–3 times weekly	Fine scrub, mask, or glycolic at 2% applied once weekly	Use delicate exfoliant (if skin is too sensitive, do not exfoliate) applied 1–2 times weekly	Exfoliating scrub, applied once weekly

MENOPAUSE MAKEOVER SKIN REGIMEN

SKIN TYPE

NORMAL	OILY	DRY	SENSITIVE	DEHYDRATED
MASK				
Apply a nourishing mask, alternating with a deep cleansing mask, 1–2 times weekly	Apply a deep cleansing mask twice weekly	Oil-based mask applied 1–2 times weekly	Apply a soothing mask once weekly	Nourishing mask, applied once weekly

SKIN CARE TIPS

- If you have combination skin, treat the T-zone area with an oily skin regimen, and outside the T-zone with either normal or dry regimes.

- If your skin is mature, treat using the dry skin-care regimen.

Tell yourself,
"I am healthy and beautiful"
five times today.

KEEPING ALL OF YOU BEAUTIFUL DURING MENOPAUSE

As we age, many of us focus on beautifying our faces, because it is the one area we can't hide. During menopause, it's time to take special care of all of you—pamper your neck, body and hands, too:

HANDS: Apply daily hand moisturizer and use SPF 15+. Hands love masks and exfoliation treatments, too.

BODY: Use shower gel and moisturize your entire body daily. Avoid harsh body scrubs.

NECK: Practice your face regimen on your neck daily.

How you age, and how you experience menopause will be different for everyone. Some women age gracefully, while others look 10 years older than their age. Lifestyle (exercise, diet, stress levels, sleep habits and sun protection), medical history, genes and how we take care of our skin will all be reflected in our skin. Your skin is the largest organ you have—take care of it.

Beyond a new skin-care routine, I discovered that accepting and loving myself was the greatest "nonsurgical" approach to enhancing beauty. After a couple years of being depressed over my new wrinkles and sagging skin, I actually started seeing the beauty in my age. When I looked in the mirror, instead of focusing on looking older, I decided I had earned every wrinkle on my face, and was damn proud of it.

MAKEOVER TIPS

- Visit your dermatologist and check moles regularly.
- Meditate. Managing stress is the first step to beauty. Stress is an instant skin destroyer.
- If you have sensitive skin, use fragrance-free and hypoallergenic products, exfoliating very little.

GETTING PROFESSIONAL HELP

Most of us are too busy to wait for over-the-counter results, and would prefer running to the dermatologist for a fast beauty fix. Before we move forward with magical solutions, I want to repeat: "Beauty radiates from a happy spirit and healthy body," not a plastic surgeon. That said, there are some relatively noninvasive procedures that can help erase some of the most common signs of aging. Even with my newfound pride in wrinkles, I, too, ran to my dermatologist for some beauty magic after watching my once-radiant skin sag, spot and drop. After years of hormone use, I had large brown spots on my face and tiny spider veins on my legs. I could live with my minor wrinkles and sagging, but the spots and veins had to go!

THE MOST COMMON SKIN COMPLAINTS ATTRIBUTED TO AGING:

Brown spots /sun damage	Dry skin	Spider veins/legs
Saggy skin	Facial veins /red spots	Droopy eyelids with crepey skin
Blotchy complexion	Hair everywhere, or disappearing hair	Rosacea
Wrinkles		

In 2008, almost 11.7 million surgical and nonsurgical cosmetic procedures were performed in the United States, according to the American Society for Aesthetic Plastic Surgery. Nonsurgical procedures make up 82 percent of the total. The most popular nonsurgical procedure is Botox, followed by hyaluronic acid fillers, laser skin resurfacing and microdermabrasion. Thirty-five- to fifty-year-olds get the majority of cosmetic treatments; this is the time in our lives when we are most self-conscious about aging.

If you decide to see a dermatologist to reverse the signs of aging, understanding your options will help you successfully choose the correct technique for your budget. Did you know there are many ways to "unwrinkle" a wrinkle? You can fill it, plump it, relax it, peel it or resurface it.

With so many options, what is a menopausal gal to do?

1. Make an appointment with a board-certified dermatologist. Get references.

2. Discuss your concerns (wrinkles, brown spots, veins).

3. Listen carefully to the doctor's suggestions. Ask these questions:

   What results can I expect?

   Do you have "before" and "after" shots of the procedure?

   How many times have you performed this procedure?

   Is my skin type correct for the suggested procedure?

   What is the recovery time?

   Are there side effects and risks?

   How long do the results last—is there follow-up work?

   How and where is the procedure performed? How long will it take?

   What will it cost?

   (Let the doctor know if you have a history of scarring or herpes—both can affect the treatment outcome.)

4. Be prepared for the procedure. Do you need to schedule recovery time (hiding time)? Can you afford it? Is the suggested procedure best for you?

5. If you need a second opinion, get one. It is *your* face!

CRASH COURSE IN NONSURGICAL TREATMENTS

Nonsurgical cosmetic treatments won't stop the aging process, but they will help hide the effects of aging. First, decide what you want to "fix"—wrinkles, brown spots, sun damage, acne, loose skin, skin texture, large pores, discoloration, rosacea, broken capillaries, spider veins, facial flushing or scars. Fortunately, science has given us many technological options to manage these skin concerns. Your next step is to choose the technique to treat the anti-aging condition that fits your time frame and budget. Here are the most common nonsurgical options.

TREATMENT OPTIONS

Lasers

Ablative laser treatments damage the skin's surface so that it can then rebuild. Lasers are used to treat wrinkles, brown spots, sun damage, acne scarring and large pores, and to tighten skin and smooth skin texture. Cost can range from $750 to $5,000 per session, and there is recovery downtime. Nonablative laser treatments do not damage the top layer of skin. These lasers are used to smooth wrinkles, tighten skin, zap brown spots, improve rosacea, eliminate broken capillaries, and remove pigmentation and scarring. Costs can range from $250 to $2,000 per session. Most dermatologists offer package deals.

What's the difference? Ablative laser treatments have longer-lasting effects, and you usually need just one treatment. But they are more expensive and the recovery takes longer. Nonablative treatments, such as radio frequency and intense pulsed light, usually require four to six sessions and have little or no downtime. Each session costs less, but you need more treatments to get the same results as the ablative treatments.

Chemical peels

There are three categories of chemical peels: light ("lunch peel"), medium (TCA peel), deep (Phenol peel). Peels work by damaging the skin's surface to induce exfoliation through the application of various chemical agents. Light peels are used to smooth dull, uneven skin; reduce the effects of sun damage; minimize the appearance of acne scars; soften fine wrinkles; and remove brown spots. There is no downtime, but you may need multiple sessions. Medium peels are used to reduce the appearance of large pores, smooth acne scars, tighten skin, soften wrinkles, lessen brown discolorations, and repair sun-damaged skin. Downtime is two to three days, and you may need multiple treatments. Deep peels are used for deeper wrinkles, wrinkling around the lips and chin area and sun damage. Downtime is one to two weeks with long-lasting results. Costs range from $200 to $900 for a light peel. Medium peels range from $1,500 to $2,500. Deep peels range from $3,500 to $5,000.

SOLUTIONS FOR BROWN SPOTS

Are you seeing spots? You are not alone. Many women get brown spots during pregnancy, while taking birth control pills or during menopause due to the reaction of hormones or medications, and the biggest offender—the sun. If you have been exposed to the sun, are taking medications and/or are going through hormone fluctuations, you have options to regain and keep your healthy glow:

1. Prevention, prevention, prevention: Use sunscreen and wear a hat outside.
2. Use skin-lightening creams (prescribed 4% hydroquinone creams; over-the-counter 2% hydroquinone creams, Porcelana and Esoterica; these options take time to show results).
3. Use a tretinoin topical (acid form of vitamin A, the generic term for the medication Retin-A). Other brand names: Rejuva-A, Retisol-A and Renova.
4. Laser therapy.
5. Intense pulsed light (IPL).
6. Chemical peels.
7. Microdermabrasion.
8. Exfoliate using a glycolic acid.
9. Eat antioxidant foods: yellow veggies, blueberries, cherries, blackberries and other fresh fruits.
10. Use antioxidant facial products.

Dermabrasion

This ablative treatment uses a small, rapidly spinning wheel with a roughened surface to remove the upper layers of skin. Dermabrasion is good for acne scars, wrinkles, brown spots and sun damage. It is long lasting, but you will need 7 to 10 days of recovery time. Costs range from $200 up.

Microdermabrasion

This ablative treatment uses diamond chips to smooth away fine lines, uneven skin, age spots and acne scars. There is no downtime, but the results are temporary. Costs range from $150 on up.

Dermal Fillers

Many women choose dermal fillers for wrinkles around the eyes, frown lines, scars and lip enhancement. The dermatologist injects the area to be treated with a product that enhances soft-tissue volume, adding extra fullness. This treatment usually lasts three to six months, depending on the product used. Costs range from $400 to $800 per session.

Relaxers

One of the most popular treatments—you probably know it as Botox—to soften wrinkles around the eyes and frown lines. Relaxers are injected under the skin and usually last three to six months. Costs range from $300 to $500 per session.

All these non-surgical options offer immediate and visible results. Since cosmetic treatments are usually elective (not medically necessary), they are rarely covered by insurance and are therefore out-of-pocket expenses. These options may give you a head start on maintaining your youthful appearance. You will need to repeat treatments to maintain the same results over a longer period. Also, be aware that these treatments can carry risks. Speak to your doctor about potential side effects. If you want additional information, Appendix C at the back of this book lists nonsurgical cosmetic treatments in chart form.

TAKING MORE DRASTIC ACTION: SURGICAL OPTIONS

If you want to erase years off your face, and can afford it, you may need to consider a surgical face-lift. These procedures are costly, have a longer healing period and incur more risks. Ask yourself, "Is looking 10 years younger worth the risks of surgery? Can I maintain my skin with nonsurgical options and practice good daily skin care?"

ERASE YEARS FROM YOUR FACE—EXFOLIATE

Every 28 days your skin renews itself, leaving a fresh layer of baby skin cells. But as we get older, this shedding process—called desquamation—slows down, leaving us with fine lines, dry areas, and an uneven skin texture. Makeup can really accentuate this dilemma.

Exfoliation stimulates new cell growth by removing the cells your body is no longer shedding. It helps your body with the desquamation process by stripping the dead epidermal cells off the outer surface of your skin, and exposing a fresh layer of living cells. It takes a few days for a noticeable amount of dead cells to accumulate. It is best to exfoliate once or twice a week. You do not want to irritate your skin or remove healthy living cells by exfoliating too much.

Exfoliation can benefit the skin on your face, as well as around your lips, neck, elbows, knees and feet. As I have gotten older, I have noticed the skin on my heels starting to crack—and the skin on my elbows seems thicker. Most of these dilemmas have improved as a result of exfoliating. For those of you who love to self-tan, exfoliation will be your best friend. It gives your skin a smooth texture, ensuring an even tan.

There are three different exfoliating methods:

- Manual: Manually scrub off the dead cells.

- Chemical: Dissolve with chemicals the gluelike substance that holds the dead cells together.

- Enzyme: Dissolve with enzymes the gluelike substance that holds the dead cells together.

They all work equally well. I was absolutely amazed at the results of administering such an inexpensive and simple process on my skin. Don't forget to exfoliate your elbows and feet; the benefits are immediate.

LOVING YOUR LOCKS

Why is it that women fuss with their hair and guys usually don't? Well, the answer is thousands of years old. In many cultures, a woman's locks represented status and sexual availability. Just as a man may strut his strength and money, a woman used her beauty—and her long, healthy hair—to attract a suitable partner. When we enter menopause and start noticing thinning hair, unwanted hair on our face, thinning eyelashes and graying hair, it is no surprise that these changes cause anxiety.

WHERE DID MY HAIR GO?

Forty to 50 percent of women report some hair loss or thinning during menopause. Thinning hair and hair loss can lower self-esteem and cause embarrassment. The most common form of female hair loss is genetic, called *androgenic alopecia* (AGA), which is the same as male-pattern baldness. Female hair loss during menopause can be caused by many different factors— genetics, age, fluctuating hormones and stress. Other, nonmenopausal medical issues can cause hair loss, too. If you're concerned that your thinning hair is due to a different condition, be sure to consult your doctor for a correct diagnosis.

COMMON REMEDIES FOR FEMALE HAIR LOSS

There are things you can do to alleviate AGA:

ROGAINE: FDA-approved, over-the-counter preparation of topical minoxidil (2%). This treatment helps to enlarge and lengthen your hair follicles, which extends the growth phase of your hair. This topical treatment does not cure hair loss, but can slow down the hair-loss process.

SUPPLEMENT YOUR NATURAL HAIR: Wigs, hairpieces or hair additions, such as hair weaves may cover up the loss of hair.

HAIR TRANSPLANT SURGERY: Transplant surgery is an option, although it is expensive, can be painful and takes up to two years to complete.

DRINK TEA: Some claim that consuming green tea helps, although this hasn't been proven.

SPECIAL SHAMPOOS: Some women find that using shampoos containing hyaluronic acid can retard hair loss, but there is no scientific evidence that this works.

WHERE HAVE MY EYELASHES GONE?

What?! No more batting your eyelashes at the cute guy next to you? Just as we can start losing hair on our heads, your eyelashes can thin as well.

The good news is there are solutions. Depending on the severity, you may consider dying your lashes. Some mascaras claim to enhance eyelash appearance. Many women have false eyelashes fitted, but make sure these do not irritate your skin, making eyelash loss worse. If you suspect that your eyelashes many be thinning because of allergies, change your eye makeup and eye cleanser. Revitalash™ is a popular eyelash conditioner that yields thicker, fuller-looking eyelashes in just four weeks. If you are dealing with health issues, discuss your thinning eyelashes with your health-care provider. There is no need to lose your luscious lashes during menopause.

WHY DO I HAVE WHISKERS?

Over 40 million women in the United States alone have unwanted facial hair. Unwanted facial hair may appear as part of the normal aging process: it may also stem from fluctuating hormones as we go through menopause. Some women may only experience a few stray hairs on the chin, while others may grow visible hair on the upper lip. A small percentage of menopausal women develop a heavy, beardlike growth called hirsutism. Whether your growth is slight or extremely obvious, facial hair can cause self-consciousness and embarrassment.

There is nothing worse than looking in the mirror and finding a black hair growing out of your chin or a mole or worse—out of your forehead. What makes this experience so disturbing is that that hair was probably growing there for the past week and everyone but you noticed it. During menopause there are a couple of causes of these unwanted facial visitors. Hormone fluctuations are one cause for increased facial hair. Women secrete both estrogens (female hormones) and androgens (male hormones, such as testosterone). As we age and enter the menopause transition, the levels of both hormones change, causing unwanted facial hair growth.

HOW DO YOU MANAGE OR TREAT UNWANTED FACIAL HAIR?

Women have been looking for ways to permanently remove hair for years. There are three different strategies to manage unwanted facial hair:

Temporary Removal	Medications	Permanent Removal
• Plucking • Bleaching • Chemical depilatories • Shaving • Waxing • Threading	• Vaniqua™ (not available in Canada)	• Laser and intense pulsed light (IPL) • Electrolysis • Hormone treatment • A birth control pill

Unwanted hair can be managed once you find a solution that works for you. Some women have great success with plucking a few stray hairs and bleaching the upper lip; others must resort to more aggressive and expensive methods to conquer unwanted hair.

BEAUTY SECRETS TO LOOK YOUR BEST

As our bodies change inside and out, we need to adapt our beauty secrets. Practicing new beauty tricks can update your image. With a new hairstyle, updated makeup and a brighter smile, you can spice up your makeover so you look and feel like a new you. I felt ten years younger after I bleached my teeth, and my completion looked more radiant using a new light-reflecting foundation. After an updated haircut and color adjustment, I felt fashionable and sassy. Waterproof mascara can save the day if you are suffering from hot flashes!

Focus on what makes you feel beautiful.

A NEW HAIRSTYLE CAN MAKE YOU LOOK AND FEEL YOUNGER

Whether you are losing your hair, or wishing it were not growing on your face, getting a new hairstyle can completely update your look. Many of us have had the same hairstyle and color for the past 10 or 20 years. What made you look hot 20 years ago will probably need revamping today. I have had the same hair color and cut most of my life. Menopause weight gain caused my face shape to become rounder, and the onset of rosacea changed my complexion tone. With warm tones woven in my hair and a new hairstyle, I felt and looked years younger. For women dealing with hair loss, a shorter style offers more volume. For those with too much hair, a longer, layered style will balance your face with your locks. Your hairstyle can completely transform your look.

HAIR COLOR

Don't fret about gray hair! If you are just getting a few gray strands, plucking is an easy and immediate solution. Or select a new hair color that is perfect for your complexion. A new hairstyle with a flattering color is a wonderful way to express your individuality, and look years younger! If you have a beautiful head of gray or silver, embrace it. Gray hair can be elegant.

How do you pick a hair color that is best for you? First, you must determine if your complexion is either "warm" or "cool" in tone. An easy way to find out is to look at the veins in your arms in natural light. If your veins look green you are warm; if they look blue you are cool.

Review the chart on the following page to confirm, and note the suggested hair colors for your category.

COOL CATEGORY	WARM CATEGORY
EYES	
Black-brown, dark-brown, dark-blue, gray-blue, hazel with white, gray or blue flecks	Golden brown, hazel with gold or brown flecks, turquoise, green-blue
HAIR	
Blue-black, ash brown, ash blonde, deep brown, platinum blonde	Red, strawberry blonde, gray-yellow, deep brown with gold or red highlights
SKIN	
Very dark brown, true olive, medium with golden undertones, pale, bronze, medium pale	Pale with golden undertones, freckled, brown with pink or golden undertones, peachy or with peachy undertones, ruddy

Updating your hairstyle and hair color is a fun and easy way to boost your self-esteem. If you are feeling insecure about your menopause midsection, a new hairstyle will bring the attention up to your face!

MENOPAUSE MAKEUP SECRETS

A few makeup tips can enhance your appearance, and make you look and feel years younger. Makeup habits that worked for you in the past may need some updating to diminish the signs of aging. Generally speaking, it's better to go for a natural look. With more natural color tones and application, you'll look fresh and healthy—and younger! There are also many anti-aging makeup products available, such as SPF makeup and anti-aging foundations packed with antioxidants. Focus on your positive features, and let your natural beauty shine through, using new makeup tips.

Foundation

- Use moisturizer before applying foundation. If you have dry skin, apply a little moisturizer to your makeup sponge, then apply foundation.

- Choose the correct color (ask an expert at the makeup counter for confirmation). Never buy foundation darker than your skin tone.

- Choose a foundation for your skin type. For oily skin, use an oil-free foundation; for dry skin, use a foundation rich in moisture.

- Purchase foundation with SPF 15+ unless you are wearing a moisturizer with SPF.

- Remember: Less foundation is better than more; too much makeup can settle in your fine lines.

- Try an illuminating or light-reflecting foundation. It will brighten your skin, and make you look years younger. These products contain microscopic particles to reflect light.

- Use a sponge to apply foundation to a clean face and neck. Apply foundation in the center of your face and blend outwards, avoiding fine lines.

- Only apply foundation where needed. Often just applying foundation to the chin, cheeks and forehead will give you coverage for a fresh look.
- Blend foundation around the chin and neck areas.
- After you have applied your foundation, rub your palms together. Then press them onto your face. The warmth from your hands not only feels good, but also softens the foundation.

- Hot-flash foundation advice: Too much foundation is unforgiving during a hot flash. There are sweatproof foundations and primers available, but the less foundation you wear the better. Carry facial blotting papers, a hand fan and touch-up foundation to freshen up after a hot-flash attack.
- Lightly mist your face with water to freshen up your makeup throughout the day.

Concealer

- Purchase a concealer with a yellow tone, lighter than your natural skin tone.
- Use the tip of your ring-finger to gently pat the concealer under the eyes and on other areas that need coverage.
- Moisturize your skin before applying concealer.

- Apply concealer from the inside of the nose, up to the lash line and on the dark areas under your eyes. Do not apply concealer on the eyelid.
- You can also use concealer on blemishes, scars and brown spots.
- There are waterproof concealers for those suffering from hot flashes.

Powder

- Avoid powder if you can. It will accentuate facial hair and wrinkles.
- If you choose to wear powder, purchase a translucent powder with a matte finish.

- If you like the matte look powder offers, plus the benefit of setting your foundation, use powder sparingly. If you suffer from hot flashes, your powdering effort may need to be repeated after every hot flash. Hot-flash sufferers should beware: The more makeup you wear, the more will sweat off during a hot flash. Less is better.

Lips

- Choose light and warm colors. Darker lipsticks accentuate problem areas and can make you look harsh.
- Line your lips with a lip pencil or lip liner before adding lipstick or lip gloss. Use a soft lip pencil with a wider tip so you can blend the lip's edges.
- Wear a lip balm with SPF 15+.

- Select natural-colored lip glosses.
- Avoid bright colors and frosted lipsticks.
- To make your lips appear fuller, you can add a touch of gloss to the inside of the bottom part of the lip.
- Use lip products with an emollient to keep lips soft. Also use lip balm to moisturize lips at night.

- If your lipstick bleeds during the day, apply powder to the lips before putting your lipstick on.

- Use a lip brush when applying lipstick.

Eyes

- Choose lighter, warm, earthy tones. Purchase eye shadows that have 2–3 tones in the palette.

- Use eye shadows with a matte finish (frosted shadows will attract light and draw attention to those wrinkles you want to disguise).

- Avoid bright colors and frosted shadows.

- Shadows are better than creams. Creams will settle in eye creases.

- Always remove eye make-up before going to bed.

- Use an eye-shadow brush to apply.

- Curl your eyelashes to open eyes. Use a lash curler just after your shower. Your lashes are easier to curl when they are warmed up after your shower.

- Once you select a color tone, work with the 2–3 colors in that palette. Darkest color goes on the eyelid crease area. Medium-color eye shadow goes on the eyelid and the lightest color goes under the eyebrow toward the outer corner of the eyebrow. Blend all the shades.

- If you have sensitive eyes, purchase hypoallergenic makeup.

- If you like to define your eyes, use eyeliner. Brown or charcoal are usually better choices than black. Waterproof eyeliners are available if you are suffering from hot flashes.

- Finish your eyes with mascara, selecting a natural color. For the first coat, apply a volumizing formula, starting from the base of your lashes. Then apply a second coat of lengthening mascara. Purchase waterproof mascara—there's no need for raccoon eyes even if you're having hot flashes!

- Keep brushes clean.

Cheeks

- Use blush to contour your face.
- Avoid bright pinks; instead, use softer browns and peaches.
- Do not use too much blush. After applying blush to your brush, tap any excess off the brush before applying.

- Avoid blush with sparkles.
- To determine where to apply blush; bend over for 30 seconds; when you stand up, note where your natural color appears on your cheeks. Apply blush in this area, and then brush and blend outward.

You don't have to be a makeup artist to find your natural beauty. If you need a second opinion, set up a makeup consultation appointment at your local department store. These professionals can offer tips and confirm the best colors for you. With all the new anti-aging products flooding the market, a professional can give you samples to try before you make a purchase.

DRESSING THE NEW YOU

There are more than 40 million women over size 14, and over 44 million women going through menopause. Shopping for a new outfit can be frustrating when your body is changing as fast as your hormones and designers are focusing on younger, smaller women.

No matter what your size or shape, there are styles to flatter your good points and minimize those areas you'd rather play down. The first step to revamping your wardrobe is to identify your shape and note the styles that flatter your shape. Then clear all the unflattering clothes you have been wearing from your closet and go shopping! Bring a friend and a list of the clothes that flatter your body type.

MAKEOVER TIPS

Update your hairstyle and color before going shopping.

WHAT TO WEAR—AND WHAT NOT

	HOURGLASS *Classic curvy with large bust and hips, and a narrower waist.*	RULER *Chest, waist, and hips are equal measurements; smaller bust.*	APPLE *Fuller in the middle.*
TOPS	Fluted sleeves. Wrap tops. Fitted jackets. Blouses with defined waistlines. V-neck, scoop necklines. Tailored tops.	Bold colors. Jackets with wide lapels and pockets that flare from waist. Strapless tops. Vests. Ruffles.	Tailored jackets with a simple flare. Tops tighter under the bustline. Wide neck or wrap tops.
BOTTOMS	A-line skirts. Flare or boot-cut pants with flat front.	Boot-cut pants. Wide-legged pants. Wear shoes with heels.	Wide-legged pants with flat front.
DRESSES	Wrap dresses. Hem at knee or midcalf, if you are tall.	Shirt dresses with breast pockets. High-waisted dresses. Wear belt over or just below waistline.	Styles that fall softly from the bustline and have a flare just below the knee.
TIPS	Emphasis on natural curves. Choose narrow clothing lines.	Create curves. Use scarves, belts, accessories.	Draw attention toward neck with scarves, accessories and rounded collars.
NO-NOS	Tucks and gathers. Bulky fabrics. Too much detail around the bust. Spaghetti straps or halter tops. Too many accessories.	Plunging necklines. Tapered pants. Boxy styles. Tight tops.	Denim jackets. Pleated pants. Shiny fabrics around belly.

TO WEAR—FOR YOUR FIGURE

	PETITE *Shorter height with narrow hips and tiny shoulders.*	**PEAR** *Upper body is smaller than your lower body, hips larger than shoulders.*	**V-SHAPED** *Shoulders are two inches wider than hips; fuller breasts, long legs.*
TOPS	Strapless tops. Focus on the waist or bust with ruffles, scarves and belts.	Tailored tops. Jackets and tops hit narrow part of waistline or midthigh. Scoop neck, V-neck, rounded or square necklines. Puffy sleeves.	Jackets that flare at hem. Shawl collars. Round or V-neck.
BOTTOMS	Boot-cut pants with high pockets.	Wraps and A-line skirts, hem at knee. Pants at waistline or just below. Boot-cut.	Skirts or pants with flare. Wear belt lower than your waistline. A-line skirts. Boot-cut pants. Hipster jeans. Fitted tops.
DRESSES	Solid colors, hem at knee.	Hem at knee. A-line dresses. Flare hem.	Hem at knee. A-line dresses.
TIPS	Dress monochromatically.	Wear darker colors on bottom, soft patterns on top.	Show-off legs. Wear sexy shoes. Wear bright colors and thicker fabrics on bottom. No scarves or bulky accessories.
NO-NOS	Shoulder pads. Long skirts. Ankle straps on shoes. Big prints.	Tight clothes. Busy patterns on bottom. Pant side pockets.	No baggy pants. No skinny jeans.

No matter what your body shape, during menopause your waistline may get larger. With body fat shifting to the belly, it's time for a shopping spree!

TWELVE STYLING TIPS

1. Wear clothes that fit; baggy clothes will only make you look bigger.

2. Measure yourself so you know what size to buy.

3. Monochromatic outfits are slimming. Dressing in one color is always flattering and classy.

4. Add color and accent with accessories, scarves, blazers or cardigans. Necklaces should be worn long. Scarves should be long and tied loosely.

5. Any stripes should be vertical.

6. If you wear a belt, it should be light and feminine. A bulky heavy belt can "shorten" you.

7. Wear a heel on your shoe. Feeling and looking taller is always a winner.

8. Choose darker colors for your basics. Navy, charcoal, gray and black are all slimming.

9. Undergarment foundations are my newest discovery this year! I purchased an all-in-one shaper so I was firmer and my soft lumpy spots didn't ruin a nice line in an outfit.

10. Know your best feature. If it is your legs, wear knee-length dresses. If it is your bust, choose a plunging neckline. Whatever your special asset, this is the time to flaunt it.

11. Carry an oversize handbag. Proportion can fool the eye. Square-shaped bags look good on rounder figures, and a purse with a strap should not land in your "problem" areas.

12. Once you update your wardrobe, add a few sexy shoes, a fun handbag and accessories for day and nighttime.

MAKEOVER TIPS

- Choose colors that flatter your skin tone.
- Dark colors minimize.
- Patterns and bright colors bring attention.
- Avoid narrow-ankle pants.
- Avoid high-waisted outfits—they'll make you look bigger in the middle or even pregnant.
- Purchase an outfit that flatters your body, not necessarily one that fits in with the latest hot trend.

UNDERGARMENTS

Spoil yourself with romantic sleepwear and undergarments. Not for "him" but for you. When I was feeling fat, frumpy and hormonal, I went out and purchased some sexy underwear and PJs. When I wore the sexy underwear, I felt like I had a little secret that no one knew about but me. I smiled all day wearing my pretty panties and felt confident that I possessed the experience and knowledge that only comes with age. And at night, I felt sassy slipping into a feminine outfit. Try it!

The correct-fitting bra can make you look perky—and 10 pounds lighter— in less than five minutes.

How to properly fit a bra

Almost 80 percent of all women are wearing the wrong-size bra. A bad-fitting bra can make you look frumpy and lumpy. One of the smallest areas of our midsection is just under our boobs. Don't hide a thinner area with droopy boobs—lift those "sisters" and show off that sexy area. Many of us have continued to wear the same-size bra for decades, despite our changing bodies. Many women have never been properly measured and fitted for the correct-size bra. With aging, your body shape may change, as well as your bra size. When we shop for bras, we hunt for styles we like, but the fit is just as important.

Size matters

It is easy to properly fit a bra. First, determine your chest size or band size (32, 34, 36, 38, etc.). Second, determine cup size (A, B, C, D, CC, DD, etc.).

{ Step 1: Band size }

Wear your best-fitting bra, and measure directly under the breast. Exhale when measuring. Round up to a whole number. If the number is even, add four inches. If the number is odd, add five inches. This is the band size.

{ Step 2: Cup size }

Stand straight. Arms at your sides. Loosely measure at the fullest part of your breast while wearing a nonpadded bra. Do not wear a sports bra during measuring. Round up numbers to a whole number.

{ Step 3: Calculate bra size }

Subtract the step-1 band measurement from the step-2 cup measurement. If there is a half-inch measurement, increase the cup one size up.

(Cup sizes: AA = no difference, A = 1", B = 2", C = 3", D = 4", DD = 5", F = 6", G = 7", H = 8")

Once you've taken your measurements, go to the lingerie department of your favorite store and try on bras with your new calculations. Don't be afraid to ask for help from the lingerie salesperson.

MANICURES AND PEDICURES—
LIFE'S LITTLE LUXURIES

As the years pass, schedules fill up and responsibilities preclude pampering time, we often forget to make time for manicures and pedicures. During your Menopause Makeover, schedule a manicure and pedicure weekly or semimonthly. It is a wonderful way to make time for yourself. Take care of your hands and feet during menopause.

This chapter is dedicated to rediscovering your beauty, inside and out. Most of us have been practicing beauty tips from our teen years that no longer work during menopause. Cleansing habits, makeup application, purchasing properly fitted bras, wearing flattering styles and personal grooming must all be updated when we go through "the change." We must change. In order to regain control of our beauty, we must embrace these changes as much as we did during our teen years.

You will increase your confidence and self-esteem with a new, hip pair of glasses or sexy jeans, or a flattering new hairstyle. Menopause and aging do not have to signal the end of feeling beautiful. Instead, you can begin to find a new kind of beauty. Let your spirit shine—that is the greatest beauty tip of all. Don't let magazine advertisements, commercials or the media define beauty for you. We are all beautiful.

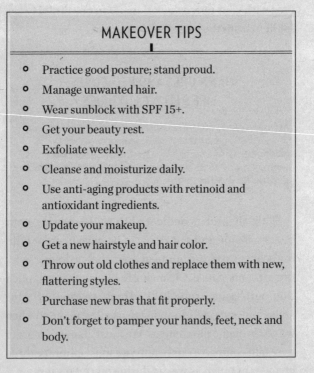

MAKEOVER TIPS

- Practice good posture; stand proud.
- Manage unwanted hair.
- Wear sunblock with SPF 15+.
- Get your beauty rest.
- Exfoliate weekly.
- Cleanse and moisturize daily.
- Use anti-aging products with retinoid and antioxidant ingredients.
- Update your makeup.
- Get a new hairstyle and hair color.
- Throw out old clothes and replace them with new, flattering styles.
- Purchase new bras that fit properly.
- Don't forget to pamper your hands, feet, neck and body.

MAKEOVER TAKE-ACTION LIST

- Update your skin-care regimen.
- Schedule a facial, and discuss skin care with the technician.
- Collect magazine clippings of hairstyles you like that you think would be good for your face shape.
- Make an appointment with your hairstylist.
- Schedule an appointment at your local department store beauty counter to discuss makeup tips and update your makeup.
- Select a teeth-whitening option.
- Buy a new, properly fitted bra and a cool pair of jeans.
- Make sure your closet has new basics and that old styles get tossed.
- Schedule a manicure and pedicure.
- Set beauty goals on pages 313 and 314.

IN YOUR ESSENTIAL PLANNER

- Track beauty goals weekly in your Weekly Progress report.
- Enter all appointments—spa, makeup artist, hairstylist—in your Month-at-a-Glance Planner to keep track of your makeover.
- Record your beauty connections in your Menopause Makeover Contacts.

chapter 6

Step Five: Am I Losing My Mind? Getting Off the Emotional Roller Coaster

We've all heard the expression *Mind over matter*. Well, going through menopause will put you to the ultimate test. With so much happening to your body and your brain, some pretty big emotions get stirred up. These changes can make you irritable, cranky, and sad—and feeling out of control over these uninvited changes. As if dealing with emotions weren't enough, my memory started to act a bit funny: Some memories came flooding back and some just seemed to disappear completely.

This chapter addresses the emotional side of menopause—the symptoms and changing brain chemistry that can affect your daily life. It is often these changes that can make experiencing menopause so challenging. Going through menopause, whether you are perimenopausal or postmenopausal, can push some big emotional buttons. Ever-changing hormones can trigger moodiness that can open the door for previously hurt feelings to surface. Other feelings pop up as a result of midlife and lifestyle changes. Throw in feelings fueled by confusing social expectations and our personal commitments, and watch out! Each section in this chapter will explain emotional challenges and offer you solutions to start feeling sane again. You'll come away with a better understanding of why you've been asking, "Have I lost my mind?"

YOUR IDENTITY

From childhood to young womanhood, each of us forms a unique identity. Women often choose between two common identifiers: marriage and motherhood and/or a professional career. We have been fortunate during the past 50 years to be able to have these choices. Now we have the choice to have children early or later in life, and can seek financial independence. When our biological clock ticks from the reproductive years into the freedom phase of menopause, we can choose to be stressed out because the baby-making chapter has ended, or we can celebrate our newly attained independence.

Menstrual cycles and childbearing involve physical transitions just as menopause does, mostly driven by hormones. It is true that nine months of uncomfortable pregnancy symptoms are shorter than five to seven perimenopausal years, but the freedom from PMS, periods, birth control and worrying about everyone else can bring relief. The journey from perimenopause to postmenopause can challenge your self-image, self-esteem and body image. This transition is a wonderful time to rethink your identity.

1. How do I define success (motherhood, career, finances, social status, relationships, community service)?

2. What dreams have I placed on the back burner, which can now be reignited?

3. What makes me happy?

4. How do I feel about age? What is my greatest fear about growing older (wrinkles, weight gain, not being sexy, health concerns)?

5. How would I rate my self-esteem (on a scale of 1 to 10, with 10 being self-confident and happy)?

6. How can I improve my self-esteem?

7. How do I rate my body image (on a scale of 1 to 10, with 10 being smoking hot)?

8. How can I improve my body image?

9. How do I view myself? How do others view me?

10. If I could change one thing about my identity, what would it be?

YOUR MOTHER'S MENOPAUSE

Many years ago, our mothers had a very different menopausal transition. Most women did not discuss their troublesome symptoms. They suffered silently, and hoped "the change" would end sooner rather than later. When I asked a friend's mother about her menopause, she said, "Oh, it was no big deal." Then her daughter quickly reminded her about her hysterectomy, and the stressful period she had experienced going through menopause. Her mother had completely blocked out her menopausal experience. Many daughters duplicate their mother's physical journey, so understanding your mother's experience—both physically and emotionally—may help you gauge your own.

Women are overwhelmed with busy schedules in our fast-paced world. Throw menopause into the mix, and we can be facing an extremely stressful time. Fortunately, a growing number of doctors and scientists in the United States today are women, and menopause research is on the rise. Menopause is finally "out of the closet."

If you can discuss menopause with your mother, it may help you navigate your own experience. It may also give your mom a chance to express buried feelings about her menopause transition.

QUESTIONS FOR MOM

1. What were your worst symptoms going through menopause?

2. Were you emotional?

3. Did you experience weight gain?

4. Did you have any medical conditions that arose during "the change"? High blood pressure? Bone density changes? Cancer?

5. How did you feel going through menopause?

6. Do you have any advice for me?

SOCIAL EXPECTATIONS

One of the biggest complaints among menopausal women is the frustration they feel from society's expectations. In the United States, as well as many European countries, women are valued for their youth and beauty. In the past, a woman's feminine beauty was considered to be *over* after menopause. No wonder our mothers did not discuss going through "the change"! Yet in other cultures, women are celebrated after they pass through menopause, and are often welcomed into the "man's world" with open arms. In Asia, women are more respected after menopause, and can achieve a higher status in society. Age is a badge of honor, not a sign of worthlessness. Sadly, in other cultures, including our Western culture, the general attitude is that menopause means a loss of beauty and youth—and that equals a loss of sexiness and value.

Yet, there is hope! And it begins with us. A few brave advertisers, Dove™ being one of them, celebrate a woman's physical passage through the different stages in her life. Almost 200,000 women a month are entering perimenopause. We can choose to be embarrassed by the experience or we can embrace the transition. We must let society know that we positively acknowledge this stage in our lives. This is the only way social beliefs, expectations and stereotypes will change—our voices must be heard. We, the baby boomers, have a loud voice. Let's use it! Then society will look at menopause as our celebration of entering into a new, liberating stage of life.

Many of us fear that men will no longer find us attractive. Men will continue to mirror our fear of aging, unless we start seeing beauty in ourselves.

HOW TO FIND YOUR MENOPAUSE SWAGGER

- Read biographies of great women who found success over the age of 40.
  I'm Not Slowing Down, by Ann Richards, former governor of Texas
  Cloris: My Autobiography, by Cloris Leachman, Oscar and nine-time Emmy Award winner
  Growing Up Again: Life, Loves, and Oh Yeah, Diabetes, by actress and activist Mary Tyler Moore
  Audition, by network diva Barbara Walters
  Age Is Just a Number: Achieve Your Dreams at Any Stage in Your Life, by Olympic gold medalist Dara Torres
  I Feel Bad About My Neck, by writer Nora Ephron
- Make a list of your life accomplishments (graduating from high school and college, marriage, children, career successes, winning a contest, travels).
- Make a list of five things you've always wanted to do (spend a week in a bungalow in Tahiti, read a Jane Austen novel, pamper yourself at a spa retreat, learn to fly or sail, write poetry, skydive). Set a goal to do or start one a month or all five over the next year.
- Every morning stand in front of the mirror naked and say, "I am beautiful and sexy." So some things are droopy and lumpy these days—don't let your self-esteem droop! Focus on your perfect self hiding under your fat suit. Firm self-esteem is stronger than a firm tush.

- Every day go out into the world knowing you are beautiful and sexy. How you feel about yourself says more to the world than your appearance.

- Find areas in your life that define you and which are not driven by your looks. What are you especially proud of? What are you especially good at? Turn off the disparaging voice in your head and write down 10 things you've accomplished that make you feel great about yourself.

- Make a list of how you could make the world a better place. Maybe you could join a volunteer organization or vow to drop groceries off for the elderly woman next door. Pick one thing from your list and go do it!

- If you had one month to live, what would you do? I doubt, it would be Botox or a tummy tuck!

- Don't let magazine ads influence your sense of self. Every time you start comparing yourself to a magazine ad, remember that the model was likely photoshopped beyond recognition!

- Treat yourself like royalty and you will feel royal. Pamper, pamper, pamper yourself. Get a pedicure, buy a new pair of shoes or take a long soak in the tub.

- Don't forget to smile.

WHAT, *ME*, CRANKY AND MOODY?

Feeling cranky, irritable, impatient and moody is common during menopause. The out-of-control and uninvited emotional outbursts are hard to live with. Some women experience higher levels of anxiety during menopause that can lead to panic attacks, dizziness and heart palpitations. These attacks can be scary to the one suffering from them, as well as to loved ones witnessing these effects. Often we can thank fluctuating hormones for our wacky emotions. Throw in hot flashes and vaginal dryness—no wonder you're cranky and moody!

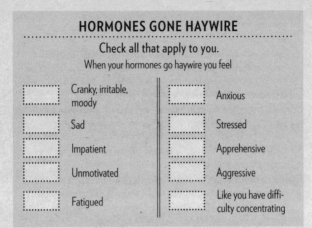

HORMONES GONE HAYWIRE

Check all that apply to you.

When your hormones go haywire you feel

☐	Cranky, irritable, moody	☐	Anxious
☐	Sad	☐	Stressed
☐	Impatient	☐	Apprehensive
☐	Unmotivated	☐	Aggressive
☐	Fatigued	☐	Like you have difficulty concentrating

When you feel cranky, list the things you are thankful for.

WHY THE ROLLER COASTER?

This menopause emotional roller coaster can happen for a variety of different reasons. Knowing the cause can help you find the solution. Speak to your practitioner if you think hormones are to blame and consider seeing a therapist if lifestyle changes have you feeling stressed. Among the factors that may be contributing to your menopausal moodiness:

- You may be suffering from hormone fluctuations. If you suffered from bad PMS due to menstrual hormones, menopause may feel like full-time PMS.

- You recently had a hysterectomy, causing your hormones to change drastically.

- You are not getting enough sleep because you're suffering from night sweats.

- You are experiencing stressful lifestyle changes, such as a career change, an empty nest, or caring for aging parents.

- You're experiencing a loss of libido.

- Life itself is stressing you out. Career stress or relationship issues can make you moody or anxious.

- You're upset at growing older. Your view of aging and menopause is negative or you feel grief at no longer being able to have children.

- Your physical health is deteriorating.

- You have a history of clinical depression; the hormonal fluctuations of menopause can trigger depressed feelings.

- You have money/ retirement fears.

HOW TO COPE

Discuss hormone therapy with your doctor, and consider the following strategies:

- Seek support from friends and family.
- Find quiet time for yourself.
- Meditate.
- Take a yoga class.
- Exercise.
- Eat healthfully (a higher-protein, low-glycemic diet).
- Avoid alcohol or sedatives.
- Discover new ways to creatively express yourself.
- Don't smoke.
- Make sure you get a good night's rest.
- Pamper yourself.

HORMONES AND THE BRAIN

The female brain goes through many changes over the course of a lifetime, largely thanks to changing levels of hormones like estrogen. In her book, *The Female Brain,* Dr. Louann Brizendine explains how the female brain changes from birth to puberty to motherhood to menopause due to changing hormones.

From birth, a girl's brain receives enormous amounts of estrogen. Dr. Brizendine says, "This high quantity of estrogen also stimulates the brain circuits that are rapidly being built…enhancing circuits and centers for observation, communication, gut feelings and caring." From the time we're little girls, estrogen is already helping us become fantastic communicators and empathizers.

Hormones play a significant role during puberty, too. Dr. Brizendine explains how fluctuating hormones affect the turbulent teen years: "The rising tide of estrogen and progesterone starts to fuel many circuits ... assuring that ... female-specific brain circuits will become even more sensitive to emotional nuance, such as approval and disapproval, acceptance and rejection. These changing circuits drive the way [a girl] thinks, feels and acts [so] a girl's primary purpose is to become sexually desirable and attractive."

When a woman is pregnant, her body produces much more progesterone and estrogen. Her brain begins to focus on nesting and her brain is calmed by progesterone. As Dr. Brizendine says, "The mommy brain is switched on right at birth by a cascade of oxytocin." Oxytocin is the maternal bonding hormone, akin to dopamine, which gives a woman those nurturing feelings. The mommy brain is committed to caregiving, putting the needs of her family over her own. Child rearing continues to be fueled by oxytocin as well as cycling estrogen, progesterone and testosterone.

Then during menopause our brains change again, as Dr. Brizendine explains, "The mommy brain unplugs. Menopause means the end of the hormones that have boosted communication circuits, emotion circuits, the drive to tend and care, and the urge to avoid conflict at all costs." During perimenopause, estrogen begins to decline, and so does oxytocin, the hormone responsible for connecting and caretaking. Menopause marks a time of low estrogen and significantly diminishing progesterone, when the brain circuits that were fueled by estrogen, progesterone and oxytocin are altered.

During menopause, a woman begins to focus on her health. During postmenopause, there is more calmness because estrogen, testosterone and oxytocin are low and steady. A woman is less emotional and becomes more interested in what *she* wants to do and less interested in taking care of others. Most women experience a shift from caregiving to personal growth from perimenopause through postmenopause.

After reading Dr. Brizendine's research, it all made sense. I wasn't losing my mind; my hormones were simply changing. Knowing that our mind chemistry changes with menopause, affecting our behavior and moods, soothed my fears. I felt validated, knowing there was a scientific reason for the way I felt.

My brain rewired from mommy brain to independent brain, no longer driven by caregiving. Of course, I still enjoy taking care of my loved ones, but it is different now. It is a choice, not an urge. What freedom! This new "menopause brain" offers us the opportunity to contribute not only to our families, but also to our communities. It can make you really feel like Wonder Woman™—you can change the world with your new menopause brain. I decided to write this book with my new menopause brain! Menopause is your time to focus on *you*.

DEPRESSION

Women who have a history of depression may also suffer from depression during menopause. Others may experience depression for the first time during the menopause transition. Depression can make going through menopausal physical and emotional changes more difficult.

Clinical depression is defined as being intensely sad or feeling severe desperation that affects your daily life for more than two weeks. Clinical depression can silently rob your life of joy, happiness and healthy relationships. If you have a history of depression, have suffered from severe PMS or postpartum depression, or have a strong family history of depression, you may be at higher risk for clinical depression. Depression is a disease caused by very real biological triggers, including declining levels of estrogen and progesterone that may disturb the levels of serotonin, medical conditions (heart disease, thyroid, sleep disorders or a head injury), and some prescription drugs.

In addition to physical causes, depression has psychological origins as well. A significant loss (a divorce, a death, new empty nest or feeling a loss of youth) can trigger depression. Situational changes that may cause depression include changes in relationships, personal losses or crises, or overwhelming situations and life changes, all of which are common to menopause.

SYMPTOMS OF DEPRESSION

- Sadness
- Hopelessness
- Feeling desperate
- Tiredness
- Irritability
- Feeling worthless
- Feeling guilty
- Feeling overly stressed about weight changes
- Loss of libido
- Changes in appetite
- Activities that used to make you happy no longer do
- Difficulty concentrating
- Sleeplessness
- Thoughts of hurting yourself

TREATMENTS FOR DEPRESSION

1. Pay attention to your moods; keep notes on how you feel in the Menopause Makeover journal.

2. Antidepressants can help alleviate depression. There are many different classes of antidepressants; most work by increasing levels of key neurotransmitters, such as serotonin, in the brain. Discuss this option, as well as other types of antidepressants, with your health-care practitioner.

3. For some women, hormone therapy has a beneficial effect when added to other antidepressant treatment.

4. Psychotherapy can help resolve many issues contributing to your depression.

5. Exercise can make you feel better. Your body creates feel-good endorphins during aerobic activity that can help improve your mood.

6. Eat healthfully.

7. Avoid excessive alcohol and caffeine.

8. Pamper yourself (get a massage, a facial, a manicure, or take a trip out of town).

9. Get enough sleep.

10. Join a support group, and surround yourself with friends and support.

Oftentimes, women suffering from depression don't even know it. If someone who loves you suggests that you get help for depression, listen!

Depression can leave you feeling lethargic and unable to properly care for yourself. If menopause is combined with clinical depression, seek help to manage your depression and other menopause symptoms. Do not go through depression alone.

MEMORY LOSS

Have you ever been out doing chores when you received a call from a friend who has been waiting an hour for your arrival, and you completely forgot? Or do you repeat yourself a few times, because you forgot you said it earlier, only to have it pointed out by your listener?

Sometimes short-term memory loss can occur when hormones fluctuate. Declining estrogen levels may affect the levels of the neurotransmitters dopamine and serotonin. A drop in these levels can lead to moodiness, fuzzy thinking and short-term memory loss. Age, stress, medications and a decline in overall health can also contribute to short-term memory loss. Also, if you are exhausted after suffering from night sweats, and not getting enough sleep, it is no surprise if you become forgetful.

You are not crazy—ask for the support of your loved ones to nurture you through your forgetful moments. Get organized with planners, calendars and PDAs. Treating night sweats and hot flashes with low-dose hormone therapy may also help you feel sharper. Keep your mind active and enjoy a healthy lifestyle. Get enough sleep; a rested mind can absorb more information.

STRESS

We all experience stress. Daily stress triggers may include relationships, children, family, finances, work deadlines, traffic, busy schedules and constantly ringing cell phones. Mix in menopause symptoms, and stress triggers can skyrocket. Hot flashes, aging, weight gain, midlife changes, empty nest, sleepless nights and a low libido can all crank up the stress meter. Just when you need to be at your best to manage all this stress, your fluctuating hormone levels may affect the mood centers in your brain, causing you to melt down. Chronic stress can wreak havoc on your overall health and happiness.

WHEN YOU ARE STRESSED OUT

- It is difficult to lose weight.
- You may experience migraines, irritable bowel syndrome, acid reflux and back and joint pain.
- You feel gloomy and tearful.
- You have a hard time concentrating.
- You are constantly irritable and cranky.
- You feel hopeless.
- Damage can be caused to your immune system, making you susceptible to infections and viruses.
- You have a harder time going through menopause.

HOW TO COPE WITH STRESS

- Identify stress triggers and resolve relationship issues.
- Try stress-relieving activities, such as yoga, meditation or tai chi.
- Regular exercise releases endorphins, making you feel better.
- Schedule fun activities.
- Make time for your friends; support is important.
- Eat healthfully—avoid a diet heavy in carbohydrates.
- Pamper yourself a little bit—take a hot bath, or treat yourself to a manicure or a massage.
- Get in touch with your spirituality (see Chapter 8).
- Get plenty of rest.
- Slow down and take time in the day for yourself.
- Find a relaxing new hobby.
- Start reading more, and watch a little less television.
- Free up your schedule—start saying "no" to others, and "yes" to you.
- Make a point of laughing every day.
- Don't always answer your cell phone.

- Make fun plans for the
  weekend.

- And if you have
  a partner, a little
  affection and intimacy
  go a long way—make
  sure *you* are satisfied.

For many of us, the menopause journey can be stressful. It's especially critical that you manage stress during menopause, so that you can take care of yourself. Once you handle stress triggers, managing menopause symptoms is possible.

Whether they are suffering from midlife issues, lifestyle changes, hormone fluctuations, social pressures or personal expectations, it is no surprise that women going through menopause are emotional! Make time daily to pamper yourself, and get enough rest. You are going through a major shift in your life. Everything you know is being altered—emotionally and physically.

If you cannot manage the emotions and stress in your life on your own, seek professional help. A therapist can help with many issues in your life, relationships or past that may need to be addressed. Your practitioner can discuss the possibility of hormone therapy or the use of antidepressants. Some people find that the herb St. John's Wort helps counteract depression and stress, but if you take St. John's Wort, be sure to inform your doctor. This herb is often not compatible with other medications, and drug interactions can be dangerous.

CALL IN THE TROOPS

One of the greatest contributions you can make to help maintain your emotional health is to seek support from loved ones, friends or a psychotherapist. Add the names and contact information of your support team in the Essential Planner on page 339.

Discuss treatment options with your doctor if you are suffering from depression, moodiness, emotional outbursts, forgetfulness and fuzzy thinking. Inform your health-care provider about any genetic predispositions, health issues and lifestyle or relationship changes.

MAKEOVER TIPS

- Let your friends and loved ones know you are struggling with uncontrollable crankiness, moodiness and fuzzy thinking; ask for their support.

- When you start feeling a surge of out-of-control emotions building up, stop, breathe, count to 10. Take a "time-out" for yourself.

- If you suspect that these crazy emotions stem from hormonal changes, discuss hormone therapy and/or antidepressants with your doctor.

- If your emotions are related to relationship or lifestyle concerns, schedule an appointment with a psychotherapist.

MAKEOVER TAKE-ACTION LIST

- Spend time reviewing your answers to the Identity Questionnaire on page 188.

- Speak to your mother about her menopause experience. See the suggested questions on page 190.

- Are you suffering from menopausal crabbiness, moodiness, depression or short-term memory loss? __ Yes __ No If yes, what solutions work for you? Refer to page 196 (how to cope with the crazy menopausal emotional roller coaster).

- What can you do to cope with your stress? Refer to page 203.

- Identify and enter goals on pages 314 and 315.

- If you already have a busy schedule, start cutting back on your responsibilities. Make time for you.

IN YOUR ESSENTIAL PLANNER

- Record any take-action tasks in your Month-at-a-Glance Planner.

- If you are suffering from any abnormal emotions, depression or short-term memory loss, schedule an appointment with your doctor or psychotherapist.

- Make a list of friends you can call for support; record their contact information on page 339.

- In your 12-Week Plan, schedule quiet time.

- In your 12-Week Plan, schedule pampering time for yourself.

- Make note of any emotional outbursts in your 12-Week Planner.

- If you are suffering from depression, memory loss or stress, document these episodes in your medical forms.

- Journal your feelings daily.

- List your support team and doctor contacts in your Menopause Makeover Contacts.

chapter 7

Step Six: Why Are They All Running Away? Strengthen Your Relationships and Get That Sizzle Back into Your Sex Life

He stood frozen like a deer caught in the headlights of a car. His eyes bugged out and the hair on the back of his neck was standing at full attention. His shoulders hunched up around his ears. He was in full retreat mode. White as a ghost and trembling with fear, he worried that one step in the wrong direction could result in his own demise, or end his marriage. How did he get here? What happened? How could he escape?

Welcome to my husband's world. While my world was consumed with daily emotional avalanches and dreadful menopause symptoms, his world was filled with confusion. Ravaged by hot flashes, weight gain, cranky moods, lack of sleep, tender breasts, disappearing self-esteem and a dry vagina, I had lost my sense of compassion and understanding. I had become an erupting volcano of anger. After a few months, I wondered, "Why is everyone running away from me?"

For most women, loved ones are one of our greatest sources of satisfaction. The majority of our adult lives have been spent caring for others, and we tend to put ourselves second to those we love. You have probably given a large part of your life to your family. During menopause, your most beloved relationships may be sorely tested.

Once you reach menopause, irritability may increase because the ratio of estrogen to testosterone in your system starts shifting. Fluctuating hormones can cause some serious crankiness. And keeping the peace no longer seems like the priority it was during your childbearing years. As our hormones change, we change emotionally, too.

So what's a menopausal soul to do? This chapter will present easy-to-understand explanations about how our changing hormones can affect our relationships, and offer some possible solutions. It also includes helpful hints for your guy and suggestions for what to say when you're in a rough spot. The Menopause Makeover can only be successful when your partner, family and friends understand what you are experiencing, so you can get the support you need.

NOTE

Acknowledging that relationships exist between women and men, and between women and women, this chapter has something for everyone. Because a female partner can have the advantage of relating to her menopausal lover differently than a man can, some of the information in this chapter is directed toward the male in the female/male relationship. Relationships with other loved ones, friends and coworkers are also addressed here.

RELATIONSHIPS AND SEXUAL HEALTH

"Honey, you are never *in the mood anymore*. It's been a while, I really need to *get some*," **he says,** staring at the ceiling in the dark.

She says, "It's always about *you*. What about me? I've been feeling like crap lately. I'm exhausted—these night sweats keep me up all night. All I do is household chores, deal with your stuff and work. Frankly, why is it always about you?"

He says, "Well, for the past 12 years, you never complained. I thought you liked to make love to me."

She says, "Even if I was up for sex, my vagina is so dry it hurts every time we do it. Do you wonder why I'm not in the mood? I'd rather go shoe shopping than make love to you."

She rolls over, pulling up the covers. **He rolls over.** Facing away from each other, she stares into the darkness, angry and misunderstood. He kicks the sheets off his feet, frustrated and disappointed.

Some studies claim that guys between the ages of 20 and 32 think about sex every 52 seconds, and women think about sex once a day. As we enter perimenopause, the female sex drive can decline significantly, continuing through postmenopause. Over 50 percent of menopausal women may experience a lower sex drive. As we age, the sexual desire gap between men and women may widen. For some women, sexual desire may increase, but this is not as common. If you want to nurture a healthy relationship, you will have to address the declining-libido issue.

Hormones can affect relationships physically and emotionally during menopause. Usually the partner in your life will notice your lack of libido before noticing that you are completely wretched from hot flashes.

When I asked a group of menopausal women between the ages of 41 and 54 if they still felt sexy during menopause, over half of them said no. I think the other half lied. The majority of women attributed their fading interest in wanting to "make whoopee" to:

- Feeling unattractive from weight gain.
- Declining libido.
- Vaginal dryness.
- Lack of sleep from night sweats and hot flashes.
- Moodiness.
- Not being happy.
- Feeling old, fear of aging.
- Being depressed.
- Being fatigued.
- Feeling isolated.
- Feeling a sense of loss at not being able to have children anymore.

How could anyone feel romantic with these all-consuming negative feelings, combined with overwhelming menopause symptoms? Most of these mood-breakers are emotional; the others are physical or situational.

PHYSICAL FACTORS THAT CAN AFFECT SEXUAL FUNCTION

- Medications, such as antidepressants, mood stabilizers, contraceptive drugs, antihistamines, sedatives, anti-hypertensives and/or medications for blood pressure or thyroid deficiency can all decrease sexual desire.
- Fluctuating hormones.
- Midlife stress, brought on by career change, relationships, loss, divorce, caring for parents and financial concerns.
- Health issues, such as heart disease or diabetes.

Approximately 47 percent of women experience sexual difficulties, according to the National Health and Social Life Survey and the Global Study of Sexual Attitudes and Behaviors, with a decrease of sexual desire being the most common.

IF YOUR LIBIDO IS DECLINING, ASK YOURSELF THESE QUESTIONS:

1. Is it physical?
   - Do you experience pain during intercourse?
   - Can you achieve orgasm?
   - Can you maintain arousal?
2. Is it lack of desire?
   - Do you desire genital contact with your partner?

○ Are you interested in sex? Do you have sexual thoughts and fantasies?

3. Is it related to your relationship satisfaction?

○ Are you happy with your relationship?

○ Does your partner please you sexually?

Many aspects may affect your libido: desire, arousal, lack of lubrication, pleasure with orgasm, pain during intercourse, lack of sexual thoughts, aversion to sexual activity, sexual frequency, lack of receptivity and relationship satisfaction. Medical conditions, such as depression, thyroid disease, androgen insufficiency, diabetes, cardiovascular disease or neurological disorders can also increase your risk of sexual dysfunction.

A variety of factors may affect sexual health: emotional, physical, cultural, medications, medical conditions, relationship satisfaction and midlife situations.

We live in a sexualized society that celebrates youth. This can leave a menopausal woman feeling frustrated and angry, self-conscious about her signs of aging or scared about no longer being in the mood for sex. Many feel embarrassed to talk about it. We are sexual beings. Paying attention to your sexuality during menopause can deepen your relationship.

FIVE STEPS TO MANAGING A DECLINING LIBIDO

There is nothing worse than wanting to feel sexy and passionate with your lover, only to have your body and mind completely put a damper on the mood. Your sex life needs some tender loving care, and if you practice these five steps, that sexy sizzle may return.

#1. Communication

If you are feeling undesirable and romance is no longer at the top of your list, the first thing you need to do is talk to your partner. As we get older, both men and women may notice a decline in their libido. It is normal for many to notice a change in sexual interest as we get older. Between the ages of 55 and 65, sexual desire may diminish for men and women. Having less sex is okay if both partners are satisfied with this change. If your partner is not OK with your declining libido, you need to address this symptom.

#2. Support

Getting support during this volatile time can strengthen your relationship, helping you emotionally and physically. It can be challenging to keep sexy feelings alive when you feel down on yourself and suffer from uncomfortable menopause symptoms. With some good old-fashioned support, trust, honesty, love and commitment to get through it together, your relationship can soar to new heights.

How do you go about making this menopause miracle of love happen? First, you must acknowledge that your partner may be absolutely clueless about your menopause symptoms and emotional outbursts. While you are suffering from many changes both physical and emotional, you will also need to be at the helm, educating your partner. This can be a difficult balancing act. Your partner must be informed so you can receive support.

The men I interviewed felt completely unprepared for their partner's menopausal transition. Most men survive their partner's monthly PMS and childbirth, but understanding these events will not necessarily give them the tools to cope with menopause. Unlike openly celebrated transitions like pregnancy, childbirth and child rearing, menopause is an occurrence in a woman's life that is still not openly discussed, making it difficult for a man to understand and support his partner's transition.

Your partner may not be prepared to face the new reality of less sex, having to support you more, helping around the house, listening better and turning on the air-conditioning. He probably does not know what to do or how to be around you during these unpredictable times. His greatest concern during your menopausal transition may be the fear of less sex. These worries are exacerbated by his own fear of getting old and possibly by his own changes in sexual function (see page 223). Understanding his fears will help the two of you communicate, so your partnership can be strengthened during menopause.

The majority of partners want to be supportive of their wives as they go through "the change," but you must let them know what you want. Do you need help around the house? Need a massage? A kiss? A snuggle? Do you want more cuddling and less sex? Need quiet time? Always remember that your partner has feelings, too, so supporting him is also important. He should listen to your experience, and he has the right to express his feelings or opinions in return.

This open communication can bring you to a deeper level of intimacy, strengthening your relationship and making your passage smoother. Map a course, including a little humor, to ensure an easier route. If you forget where you put the keys and he is the one who usually forgets, have fun with it. Now it is his turn to "Go find the keys!" Or better yet, when you have hot flashes, ask him to turn on the air-conditioning and bring you a cool towel. Men love a mission. Make *you* his new mission, and make sure you reward him for pampering you.

If you are going through a seriously irritable stage, nothing makes you happy and you are pissed off most of the time, give your partner warning. If he knows there is nothing he can do and you prefer to be alone, he can back off and give you space. Everyone will be happier. The more your partner knows about your experience, both emotionally and physically, the more he can be there for you as you need him. Ultimately, most guys want their women to be happy.

#3. Counseling

If you have a partner who does not support you, or is not willing to communicate, or if you yourself are struggling to communicate, it is time to seriously look at your relationship. Consider professional counseling.

#4. Adjust lovemaking activities

You may wish to consider new lovemaking activities. Allow more time for mental and manual stimulation. Remember the old days when you and your partner spent hours kissing and making love? Throw in a massage. Discuss sexual fantasies. Try a little afternoon delight in a new location; changing the time of day you engage in sexual activity and the location can add excitement. Reactivate the mind and heart. A little extra attention can reawaken a declining libido.

Sexual intercourse is not the only act in town. Oral sex is an intimate act that can allow you to have a great orgasm without the pain of sexual intercourse. You are entering a new world—be imaginative. Perhaps a new vibrating sex toy could be a fun companion. Add new sexual positions. Or "You show me and I'll show you," both learning something new about each other's pleasure. Feeling connected with your partner through the act of lovemaking can keep the passion alive and help facilitate the return of your feeling sexy. A little effort can make all the difference in your sex life.

#5. Discuss options with your practitioner

If your fluctuating hormones are indeed affecting your libido, there are therapies available. See Chapter 2 for more information.

LOW LIBIDO CHECKLIST

Discuss with your health-care practitioner:

- Your sexual history
- Any major life changes

- Your relationship—are you still attracted to your partner? Are you in a healthy relationship?

- Your medications
- Your health

HOW TO BOOST YOUR LIBIDO

If the flame of lust still lies dormant after you have communicated with your partner, reached out for support, taken advantage of counseling and adjusted lovemaking activities, it may be time to discuss other options, both hormonal and nonhormonal, with your health-care provider. A small adjustment can boost your libido.

ANDROGEN THERAPY

Many think androgens are a male hormone—but don't underestimate the power they have in a woman's body. Androgens are produced in the ovaries, the adrenal glands and the fat cells, and their role is to be converted to estrogen, as well as to stimulate sexual desire and help prevent bone loss.

It helps to think of androgens as a team composed of hormone players. There are two primary androgens—testosterone and androstenedione—and a few coplayers—DHT (dihydrotestosterone), DHEA (dehydroepiandrosterone) and DHEA-S (DHEA sulfate). If androgen levels are too high, it can cause excessive hair growth (hirsutism), acne and thinning hair. Too low and you may feel fatigued and lose your sex drive.

Androgens decrease with age, and there is no sudden change during menopause. But by the time we reach menopause our androgen levels have declined 50–60 percent. The exception is surgical menopause. Androgen excess or deficiency is common during menopause and can wreak havoc on your well-being.

When women notice that their sex drive is diminishing, many seek out a prescription from their doctor for a dose of testosterone (DHEA) thinking that will fix the problem. The use of testosterone to treat a diminished libido is still controversial. The FDA has not approved testosterone therapies for women suffering from a declining libido, but there have been both preliminary scientific studies and extensive anecdotal reports that support the use of this therapy for improving the libido. Women who are on testosterone therapy should be monitored for increased lipids, excessive hair (hirsutism) and acne.

Possible testosterone benefits

- Increased energy levels.
- Increased sexual interest.
- Enhanced orgasm.
- Increased bone density.
- May give you a sense of well-being.
- Helps build lean muscle.
- Helps deal with hot flashes.
- Enhanced short-term memory.
- Increased skin elasticity.

The downside to testosterone therapy

- Increased cholesterol and unhealthy lipid levels.
- Excessive facial or body hair.
- Deeper voice.
- Acne.
- Weight gain.
- Clitoral enlargement.
- Changes in emotions, especially increased anger.
- Being oversexed—no joke, this happens.

Many pharmacies can custom-compound a preparation of transdermal micronized testosterone 2 % (cream or ointment). A little compounded testosterone gel may be worth considering, but keep in mind that it has not been FDA-approved to treat a declining libido and long-term safety data is lacking. As with all compounded formulations, there is no quality control in the preparation and dosing may be inconsistent. Currently, there are transdermal applications of testosterone in development (sprays, lotions and a vaginal ring).

Estratest HS is a common estrogen-testosterone combination pill marketed in the United States, although it is technically only approved for hot flashes and not for sexual problems. In Canada, there is an oral testosterone off-label (not government-approved) prescription drug used by women, called Andriol™ (testosterone undecanoate).

The sophisticated orchestration of your hormones, your libido and your relationship is complicated. Insist on good communication with both your clinician and your partner. I personally discovered that my sex drive improved when I started hormone therapy.

If vaginal dryness is your only menopausal complaint, and you need only to treat the vagina, you can use low-dose vaginal estrogen in the forms of cream or vaginal suppositories to help improve lubrication. This form of low-dose estrogen does not stimulate the uterus and can generally be used safely and without the need for progesterone pills. If you have a host of other menopausal symptoms, including vaginal dryness, low-dose oral hormone therapy can likely bring relief.

Discuss your sexual concerns with your partner. There is nothing worse than lying in bed freaking out, feeling guilty and inadequate that your vagina is not lubricating as your partner is jumping through hoops to please you. Using lubricants or vaginal creams can help maintain your vaginal health and libido. Vaginal health can be improved. Communicate with your partner about your physical and emotional concerns regarding sex. Accept that your body is changing, and understand that options are available.

THE SECRET MEN DON'T WANT US TO KNOW

Men are worried that their wives will no longer be interested in sex as they age and go through menopause, but a man's sexual life changes with age, too! Men may start to notice a difference in erections. Starting around the age of 40, some men need more stimulation to get an erection.

I have had a number of girlfriends confess that their partners (after midlife) had a hard time getting erect; and when they did, it was a bit soft, did not last as long,

the ejaculation was not forceful, and it took longer to reach orgasm. I was shocked at hearing this news!

When it comes to sexuality, men go through physical and emotional changes as well. Perhaps, witnessing our changes in sexuality is a reminder of their own deceleration. We may need a shot of lubrication, but our man could be facing sexual challenges he never expected. This will affect you, too, so now is a good time to nurture a loving, sexual relationship. The communicating habits you create now will come in handy when your man begins to experience natural changes in his sexuality.

RELATIONSHIP REHAB

As if dealing with your partner weren't enough during an already overwhelming time in your life, what about the other people in your life? Just as you have to communicate with your partner, you may need to have a heart-to-heart with other people in your life. It is unfortunate that our society does not prepare us, nor the ones we love, for menopause. There are no "hot-flash seminars" or "cranky retreats" for menopausal gals.

THE GUY'S GUIDE TO UNDERSTANDING MENOPAUSE

There are a lot of different ways your partner can handle your menopause transition—some more helpful than others! If you are in a healthy relationship, most men will likely ask, "What can I do to help?" After all, when *you* are happy, *he* is happy. Men just want to know what *action*

they need to take, so they can be there for you. Most do not want to buy a book and read about it—you must tell them. They want to support you and survive your experience with as little effort and damage as possible.

On the next page is a survival list to share with your partner—it's like his menopause cheat sheet to use in case of emergency!

YOU . . . AND YOUR INNER SELF

As you develop a new relationship with yourself during menopause, you will have the wonderful opportunity to strengthen your current relationships, reconsider unhealthy relationships and ultimately create the love you want in your life. You are at the helm of your relationships. Going through the menopause journey can stimulate internal growth, embracing a future with loving relationships. It can also instigate a little spring cleaning in matters of the heart. Only you can determine if your "change" propels your life in a better direction. Women who have a loving relationship often have a smoother journey through menopause.

SURVIVAL TIPS FOR HIM

- Listen to her; don't criticize or try to fix her.
- Go with the flow; be prepared for constant mood swings.
- Be compassionate, and validate her experience (that means agree with her, don't try to fix her).
- Tell your wife that she can count on you—and mean it.
- Cuddle more.
- Tell her she is beautiful.
- Appreciate her.
- Make time for the two of you.
- Keep romance alive.

- Surprise her with flowers for no reason at all.
- Understand her symptoms.
- Support her treatment choices.
- If she is having difficulty coming to grips with her own experience, encourage her to visit her doctor and develop a network of girl-friends.
- Don't pursue sex if she is not in the mood; her body is changing.
- Don't think that her low libido or dry vagina is a reflection on your lovemaking skills.
- Don't ignore her hot flashes or night sweats. Offer to turn on the AC or buy her a little fan.

- If she's moody or cranky, offer support.
- As she is pigging out on junk food, don't tell her how fat she's getting. Really, don't.
- Surprise her with a date at the spa. Both of you can enjoy pampering.
- Tell her she is as beautiful as the day you met her. Let her know that beauty isn't defined by age.
- If she's acting depressed, offer your support. Encourage her to seek professional help if she needs it.
- If all else fails, disappear: Step out for the afternoon or give her some space. Only do this after you have tried all the above tips.

SURVIVAL TIPS FOR EVERYONE ELSE

So what about everyone else? Friends, family and coworkers need to survive your transition, too.

- Inform your loved ones that you are going through changes emotionally and physically.
- Invite them to boost your self-esteem with compliments.
- Warn them if they notice changes, from crankiness to depression, that you would appreciate some TLC.

- Request lots of hugs.
- Suggest that trying to fix you would not be a good strategy.
- Encourage open communica-tion.

MAKEOVER TIPS

- Communicate with your partner, so he or she understands your symptoms.

- Visit your clinician to discuss a declining libido and any issues with vaginal dryness.

- Don't let society make you feel inadequate about going through menopause.

- If your libido is low, discuss your treatment options with your partner and your health-care practitioner.

- Communicate with loved ones and ask for support.

- Make time for romance with your partner; feeling connected during this time can make your transition smoother. Give yourself permission to spend the night cuddling if you are not "in the mood."

- Try new lovemaking routines with your partner; use a little creativity to spice up your sex life.

- Manage your menopause as a team. If your partner was there for you during childbirth, why not during menopause? Men love to solve problems— let him be there for you. Use the "Survival Tips for Him" (page 225).

- Purchase bioadhesive lubricant if you are suffering from vaginal dryness.

- Keep a sense of humor.

- Eat healthfully, exercise and start loving your body during this powerful passage in your life.

GOOD NEWS: IF THEY RUN AWAY, THEY CAN ALWAYS RUN BACK!

MAKEOVER TAKE-ACTION LIST

- Buy bioadhesive lubricant, if needed.

- Tape the "Survival Tips for Him" on your master bathroom mirror or his toolbox, so he can use it for quick reference in case of emergency. Having it in the bathroom offers privacy, and may open the door for conversation about your experience and his.

- Record relationship goals on pages 316 and 317.

- Select one friend, family member or coworker and share your current journey through menopause; ask for support if you need it.

- If you are struggling with midlife issues, and your declining sex interest is the result of outside stress (divorce, empty nest, death of a family member, financial changes), schedule an appointment with a counselor.

IN YOUR ESSENTIAL PLANNER

- Schedule at least one night per week of intimacy time with your partner in your Month-at-a-Glance Planner. You go, girl! If you don't use it, you may lose it!

- Record your feelings in your journal.

- Schedule an appointment with your health-care provider to discuss your libido and any dry vagina symptoms. Record doctor appointments in your Month-at-a-Glance Planner.

- Document any changes in libido or vaginal dryness in your Medical Forms.

chapter 8

Step Seven: Embracing Spirituality: What You Believe Can Change Your Experience

When you feel as if you have lost control of your health, beauty, relationships, career and purpose in life during the menopause journey, spirituality is sometimes the only thing left holding you up. How you choose to live life is often influenced by your spirituality. For one person, getting fired from a job seems like the ultimate tragedy. For another, it is an opportunity for growth. A lot depends on how you interpret events in your life. Your spiritual community can be an enormous source of support during menopause.

This chapter includes suggestions that can be applied to any spiritual belief system. Prayer, meditation and giving thanks can nourish your spirituality, bringing a new perspective to your experience. Embracing spirituality during menopause can enrich your life and benefit your health.

WHAT YOU BELIEVE CAN CHANGE
YOUR EXPERIENCE

The last seven chapters have addressed serious physical aspects in the management of menopause. Yet I found that invisible thing we call spirituality to be one of the greatest sources of support during my passage through menopause. It is our nature as human beings to interpret the meaning and purpose of life. Thus, when we have a strong spiritual foundation, we have the ability to transcend many physical ailments. Being involved with a community that shares beliefs similar to your own can offer you support during menopause. It has been proven that people who have a strong sense of spirituality suffer less from hypertension, have better mental health, enjoy healthier lifestyles and actually live longer. Your spirituality can help define your menopause experience. Does menopause mean the loss of youth, beauty and childbearing years? Or does it represent a new beginning, focusing energy on your power to contribute to the community and personal growth?

Spirituality can mean different things to different people. In this chapter, I will refer to *spirituality* as the ultimate nature and purpose of our existence. Religions offer many people their source of spirituality. Others find it while enjoying a sunset, hiking or listening to music. Spirituality can offer hope and inner peace, profoundly affecting your physical and mental health and the overall quality of your life. Spirituality can be a wonderful tool, building good coping skills for managing stress and offering a sense of well-being. The power of positive thinking can even prevent some health problems. Spirituality can be an asset to good health. What you believe can change your experience of menopause.

HOW MENOPAUSE CAN ENRICH YOUR SPIRITUALITY

Going through the menopause transition can stimulate growth—personal, physical and emotional. You are not only experiencing midlife changes (children moving out, shifting relationships, finances, career, family and health), you are traveling through this transition with menopausal symptoms. Many women feel that menopause represents the loss of fertility and youth. Suffering from feelings of loss and stress can make managing menopause more challenging.

It can be tough to redefine your purpose in life when you're enduring daily doses of hot flashes, dry itchy skin and an ever-expanding waistline. Menopause will force you to make choices. You can choose to view this time in your life as exciting and full of new possibilities. Or you can bitch about it and feel sorry for yourself.

I sat around complaining about each irritating symptom and gaining more and more weight as I stuffed my face with ice cream. Understandably, many in my circle of friends and family ran away, leaving me isolated in the lowest emotional valley of my life. During this time, it was my spirituality that gave me the boost I needed to continue my climb up "Menopause Mountain." My spiritual journey changed my menopause experience. And balancing my hormones, switching to a good diet and exercising daily sealed the deal. Marching through menopause forced me to ask myself some big life questions:

Who am I?

What do I need to be happy?

What are my passions, talents and skills?

What is my purpose in life?

How do I contribute to society?

I was overwhelmed trying to answer these questions. After a few days squirming with this task, I developed a series of questions that took me on a spiritual path that helped me discover the answers for myself.

Find a quiet, comfortable place with paper and pen, clear your mind, breathe deeply, relax and express your inner self during this exercise. Just let the words and thoughts flow.

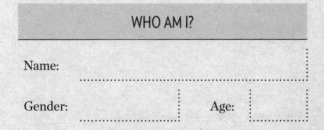

WHO AM I?

Name:

Gender: Age:

Family position in life
(mother, daughter,
grandmother, aunt,
niece):
....

Career position in life:
....

Religion or spiritual
preference:
....

How have you defined yourself through your life
experiences? (Did you graduate from college,
marry, remain single, have children, travel, win a
big contest, have an important event in your life
that defined you?)

What makes you different from everyone else
around you?

What are your wonderful qualities?

What are your less flattering qualities?

....

What is unique about you?

....

What do you value most in life?

....

How do you express yourself?

....

How do you think differently than others?
(Do you see life through political eyes? Do you see
the positive or negative in life? Do you always want
to please people? Do you naturally think things will
work out or not?)

....

Are you passionate about something special to you?

Study your answers. In one sentence answer the question, **Who am I?**

What do I need to be happy?

List all the things you need to be happy in life—go for it here.

What are my passions, talents and skills?

List your talents/skills—everything you are naturally good at and everything you are passionate about, even if you are not good at it.

What is my purpose in life?
The answer to this question will help bring clarity
to your daily life.
Why am I here?

Ask a close friend or family member what they
think your purpose is in life.

How do I contribute to society?
Review all your answers above. Is there an area that
defines you, brings you happiness or in which you
excel at that you can share with others and that will
make a difference?

After answering these questions you may choose to set new life goals during your Menopause Makeover. Do you want to go back to work? Are you ready to retire? Would you like to volunteer at a favorite organization? Have you always wanted to do something but never had the time or courage to do it? Start a new business? Go back to school? Learn a new language? Move to another location? Travel? Is it time to find new passions and give an unrealized dream attention?

Going through menopause can give you the opportunity for spiritual growth by redefining who you are, your purpose and what makes you happy; enabling you to develop new skills and passions; and determining how you want to contribute to society.

After answering the above questions I had a better understanding of myself, with a new purpose no longer defined by youth and childbearing abilities, giving me something I had never felt before. Freedom. I now had the freedom to redefine myself. This can help you connect to your spirituality. Most of us have been so busy caring for others that we have had no time left to focus on our own powerful potential. It was exhilarating and liberating to focus on the *me* in menopause...*me*—no—pause. Having wandered away from my spiritual side as I became entangled in the confusion that accompanied menopause, eventually I discovered that menopause could enrich my spirituality!

My strong spiritual foundation helped me chart my way and successfully navigate the rough seas of miserable symptoms. The menopause/midlife combo is a wonderful opportunity to reinvent yourself, creating a life that embraces your uniqueness to contribute and make a difference. The expectation to reproduce is off your shoulders. Many people still believe it is an "end" once you reach menopause. The truth is, it is a new beginning, a new chance to define your purpose outside of your biological ability to have children.

Menopause is also a perfect time to heal the past. Now is the time to address any unresolved issues. In most religions and spiritual teachings, forgiveness can be a way to help you move forward. If you are dealing with a complex situation, seek professional help. Attending to past hurts can set you free to build a life, painting a new future with a clean canvas.

Those of us going through the menopause journey have the incredible task of paving the way for our daughters. I have faith in the possibility that one day our society can fully accept this natural passage for women, and embrace it as a sacred event. How we interpret our menopause experience is the first step to that possibility. Tap into your spirituality to find your power and strength.

Where does your source of spirituality come from?

How can spirituality support your menopause experience?

THE POWER OF PRAYER AND MEDITATION

Can prayer and meditation promote good health? For thousands of years people have used prayer and/or meditation for health reasons, both for their own health and the health of others. People have formed prayer groups to pray for someone's recovery. Others have meditated privately or in groups, focusing on the health of an individual, group or the planet. There is research that claims that meditation can decrease blood pressure, relax muscles, reduce oxygen intake and lower stress hormones for hours after meditation practice.

Prayer and meditation have been a part of my life since childhood—sometimes a big part, sometimes less. With a Catholic upbringing, I found comfort in the Lord's Prayer. When I grew up and traveled the world, I witnessed the beautiful aspects of other religions. Now I incorporate meditation as a tool to tap into my inner peace. I don't do either enough; but when I do pray or meditate, I feel grounded. Both prayer and meditation bring me serenity over my usually overactive mind. During menopause it can soothe many miserable symptoms, from anxiety to hot flashes to weight gain aggravated by stress hormones.

Millions and millions of people rely on prayer and meditation to stay healthy and to return to health.

> Do something kind for someone,
> without anyone finding out it was you.

MIND-BODY BENEFITS OF MEDITATION

- Slows the progression of disease, and diminishes stress.
- Lowers blood pressure.
- Reduces elevated cortisol levels caused by stress.
- Eases chronic pain.
- Relaxes muscles.
- Brings a sense of well-being.

Prayer and meditation can bring inner peace, resulting in a sense of freedom. Both prayer and meditation focus your attention away from the beehive of thoughts in your brain. These ancient practices help make people healthier and happier. Some claim that prayer and meditation can help extend life, slowing the effects of brain aging and improving memory. It has been proven that meditation, practiced for a long period, can actually alter brain-wave patterns. This can reduce stress levels, balance emotions and provide a sense of calm. During menopause this is an excellent prescription to help regain your health and build strong self-esteem.

HOW TO MEDITATE

o Find a comfortable, quiet spot where you can sit or lie down for at least 20 minutes uninterrupted (no music or phones).

o Adjust the temperature, so you are comfortable.

o Wear loose clothing.

o Set a timer for 20 minutes, so you don't obsess over time. Select a timer with a calming buzzer.

o If you sit, try to sit cross-legged with a straight back. If that is not possible, sit in a straight-back chair. If you lie down, open your arms and legs shoulder- and hip-width apart.

o Close your eyes halfway or find a relaxed, closed position for your eyes.

o Breathe through your nose, not your mouth.

o Breathe from your belly, not your chest.

o Take full, deep inhalations and exhale slowly.

o Relax your muscles.

o Don't have expectations. Be in the present moment.

o Many people use a personal mantra to meditate (a positive phrase declaring what they want to achieve) or count their breaths (1 to 10, then repeat).

TRY THESE USEFUL PERSONAL MANTRAS:

I am healthy.

I am strong.

I am lovable.

I honor my body.

May all be happy.

I have a happy marriage.

I am beautiful.

Abundance flows into my life.

- When your mind becomes busy with thoughts, refocus on your personal mantra, or breaths (you can also use a phrase from the *Menopause Prayer or A Woman's Prayer* on pages 245 and 246).

- After you have trained your mind to focus on your mantra, or counting of breaths, begin to focus on nothing at all! True silence of the mind is the ultimate goal.

- Meditation requires patience. It is okay to have "monkey brain" (busy thinking) sometimes; mastering this is a normal part of the meditation practice.

- Do not meditate after a meal, or you may fall asleep.

PRAYERS

Feeling vulnerable and lonely during my menopause journey, I searched for an inspiring prayer. Not being able to find one I liked, I decided to write my own prayer to help give me strength during this transition.

An interesting thing happened when I began to write my personal menopause prayer—the words flew onto my computer screen as if something bigger than myself were creating this prayer. Twenty minutes later I not only had the prayer I needed, but I had two prayers. These prayers helped me in my darkest menopause times. When I read them in silence or out loud, I felt strength and hope that I would get through menopause a better person.

No matter what your spiritual preference, as women we often find comfort and peace in words. You can call these words a prayer, a poem, a short story or a mantra. Being brought up Catholic, I find comfort in the word *Lord*. To me the Lord is something bigger than me, yet the Lord also refers to that something special deep inside. Whatever your spiritual practice, feel free to use one or both prayers. You may wish to omit the word *Lord* in the Woman's Prayer if that makes you feel more connected to the message. Honor your spiritual path.

Now I share my menopause prayers with you. I hope you find comfort in them, too.

{ menopause prayer }

*Give me strength to see the beauty in womanhood
to embrace my passage from the giving of life
to the giving of myself.*

*Show me my special purpose,
releasing my spirit from expectations.*

Open my heart to love, so I may nourish my soul.

*Bring light into my darkness,
so I may see that you shine eternally.*

Hold my hand, so I am not alone.

Give me hope to see a bright future.

Shower me with patience to understand.

Wrap me with courage to celebrate my choices.

Shelter me from fear. Help me honor my body.

*Quiet my raging emotions. Cool my ever-changing body
temperature. Steady me with your strength.*

Lift me up to see beauty in my life, not in my face.

Remind me that I am desirable.

Empower me to see the good in everyone.

Open my eyes to appreciate my abundance.

Set my spirit free, so I may find my true calling.

Watch over me, so my soul may flourish.

May I find a sanctuary in your everlasting love.

{ a woman's prayer }

Lord grant me:
Serenity to accept my changes
Power to focus on the positive
Trust that I will receive support
Harmony in my emerging self

Lord grant me:
Self-acceptance in my beauty
Abundance of love
Freedom to dream
Balance to honor myself

Lord grant me:
Healing to resolve the past
The ability to manifest new beginnings
The strength to surrender
Moments to celebrate

Lord grant me:
Courage to forgive
Gratefulness for my gifts
Patience to understand that "change"
is a blessing wrapped in your love.

Just as I wrote these prayers to help me through tough menopausal times, you, too, may wish to write your own prayer. It is very therapeutic.

How to write a personal menopause prayer

- Find a quiet room.
- Make sure there are no distractions.
- Sit down with pen and paper, or in front of your computer.
- Clear your mind.
- Let go of your expectations.
- Close your eyes to connect with your inner self.
- Ask yourself, "What wisdom do I need to receive today?"
- Take a few deep breaths.

- Just start writing/ typing.
- Let the words flow— don't judge yourself.
- It's okay to cry during this experience. You are giving your spirit a place to express itself.
- When the words stop flowing, read your prayer.
- Refer to this prayer when you feel lonely, sad, frustrated, angry or lost.

CELEBRATE THE CHANGE

Now that your spiritual energy is flowing, let's harness that power so you can go through "the change" celebrated! Why is it we celebrate childbirth, despite the physical pain? Why do we celebrate a wedding, even though it usually causes great stress? Society has taught us to look at these transitions in life as a celebration, whether they were pleasant or not. Perhaps as a way to bring order to civilization, or to bring a sense of peace, so people could find joy in the changes of life. Knowing this little fact of life, let's ask ourselves, "Why can't we go through menopause celebrated, too?" The answer: We can! We can change the way society views menopause when *we* decide to celebrate our transition. If we continue to cling to youth, we cannot embrace the wisdom of aging. So how do we go through "the change" celebrated? We *choose* to go through "the change" celebrated! We must practice this celebration daily, despite frustrating symptoms and challenging midlife changes. It is your choice. If you look at menopause as a passage to be celebrated, so will others.

HOW TO CELEBRATE MENOPAUSE

- Write 3 reasons to celebrate menopause (come on now, I know you can find a few reasons).
- Read this list every day—once in the morning, and once before going to bed.
- Pray or meditate every day for support to be strong during this transition, because on the other side of menopause are new possibilities.

- Tell your loved ones and friends that you have made a choice to celebrate your passage.
- Think about this passage in your life as a positive experience.
- Embrace the many stages of womanhood. Each stage is a contribution to humankind.
- Pamper yourself—you are celebrating the new you.

MAKEOVER TIPS

- Nurture your spirituality. Read, pray, meditate, go on a spiritual retreat.

- Take care of your body. Be still, get rest and make time for pampering.

- Expand your mind. Join a spiritual group; read inspirational books and articles.

- Look at your career or consider working/ volunteering again. Find situations that can bring you joy. Start your own business. Write a book. Finish that scrapbook you started years ago.

- Go back to school. Do you have unrealized dreams? Are you curious to learn something new? Find a new passion.

- Travel. Visit the places in your dreams.

- Start a diary focusing on what you feel, not what you do.

- Make time every day to practice your spirituality. Pray, meditate, read, join support groups, volunteer, take a walk, attend spiritual services, enjoy quiet time.

- Remember to laugh.

- Choose to spend time with those with whom you share a healthy relationship.

MAKEOVER TAKE-ACTION LIST

- Record your spiritual goals on pages 317-320.
- Nourish spirituality in your life.
- Add prayer and/or meditation to your daily routine.
- Answer the "big" questions on pages 233-237.
- In a peaceful setting, read aloud the *Menopause Prayer* or *A Woman's Prayer* at least once a week.
- Write your own personal menopause prayer.
- Twice a day say, "I have a choice to go through 'the change' celebrated."
- Schedule time so you can embrace spirituality daily.

IN YOUR ESSENTIAL PLANNER

- Add daily spiritual goals to your Month-at-a-Glance Planner.
- Write daily in your journal.

chapter 9

Step Eight: Creating Happiness:
How to Be Happy During "The Change"

Was I happy about going through menopause? Was I happy about miserable menopause symptoms? Was I happy getting fat and cranky? Was I happy living with hot flashes? Was I happy living with the air conditioner on full blast in the winter? Was I happy? *Happy?* What was there to be happy about? I was miserable and pissed off that everything in my life was changing. I had to change my blouse after every hot flash. I had to change the way I ate. I had to change the way I took care of my skin. I had to change the way I had sex with my husband. Everything was changing, and I was not happy about it. How does anyone find happiness going through all these physical and emotional changes?

Webster's New World Dictionary defines *happiness* as "a feeling of pleasure, contentment or joy." This can be very difficult to achieve during the menopause journey. An avalanche of miserable symptoms and midlife changes can suffocate any hope of feeling happy.

This chapter is dedicated to digging out those happy feelings and unearthing coping skills to restore balance and joy. Once you embrace change, happiness is possible.

HOW HAPPY ARE YOU?

You would think answering this question would be easy, but it's more complicated than you might think. Imagine happiness like a pie made up of many slices, including health, career, self-esteem and relationships. When each slice of the pie is full and intact, the entire happiness pie is complete and you will feel fulfilled. If any one piece of the pie is missing, it will affect the pie as a whole: if your health is failing, your ability to work could be compromised; if you don't have strong self-esteem, your love life may suffer; if money is missing in your life, your health and self-esteem may deteriorate. When we find a balance in all areas of our life, happiness is almost always guaranteed.

So, are you happy? Let's rate the different areas of your life. Be honest—the only way to grow happier is to recognize those areas that you need to work on. This is a great opportunity to achieve high levels of happiness. Only when you're happy, will you be able to live to your full potential.

HAPPINESS QUESTIONNAIRE

Rate each category 1 to 10 (10 = over-the-moon happy, 1 = not happy at all)

[ ]	Health	[ ]	Relatives
[ ]	Love (with some-one special)	[ ]	Children
[ ]	Spirituality	[ ]	Home
[ ]	Self-esteem	[ ]	Travel/adventure
[ ]	Work	[ ]	Education/learning
[ ]	Money (Do you have enough?)	[ ]	Neighborhood
[ ]	Hobbies	[ ]	Giving
[ ]	Friends	[ ]	Creativity

SCORE RESULTS

128-260 : You are living life to the fullest, embracing the positive. You are creating your world from a place of love and joy. Start sharing your secret with others!

96-127 : You have successfully focused on some aspects of your life, but are not living in balance with others. Direct your attention with intention to one new area per week. Set goals to grow, and be open to possibilities within the areas of your life that are not yet satisfying. Continue to foster the areas giving you pleasure. Give thanks for all that you have.

SCORE RESULTS

64–95	You are below average on the happiness scale. Ask yourself what's keeping you from being as happy as possible. Make a list of things in your life that cause you unhappiness. Are there solutions? If you cannot find resolution to these areas, ask for help—personal or professional. Look at the areas of your life that bring happiness. Can you create positive change? Accept and love yourself.
32–63	You probably have situations in your life that are keeping you from being happy. How can you achieve happiness in the areas you can control? Make a list of the things that make you happy. Nourish these areas. In the areas that seem hopeless, reach out for help. Visualize happiness in all areas of your life. Pray or meditate for happiness and gratitude. Embrace your potential in all areas of your life.
0–31	You may not feel happiness is achievable, or may not have learned skills to be happy. Start seeing the positive in your life. Take control of areas that appear hopeless. Appreciate the few things in your life that bring you joy. Build on those areas. Once your happiness level grows, expand to other areas. Decide to be happy. Happiness needs to be nourished.

How do you feel about your level of happiness? What's incredible about this process is that life is always changing, so your level of happiness will change, too.

I do this exercise every New Year's Eve. Five years ago I had a great career, but no love. After looking at this situation, it dawned on me that I was working long hours so I had no time for love. After finding a balance in these two areas, I now have a great love and a new career I love, too! I focused on the area that was not fulfilled and took action. I had to look at the whole picture so I could make changes. Consider these questions:

- What areas in your life need attention?
- Is there an action you can take to initiate positive change?
- Is there a pattern of areas that are not fulfilled and areas that are making you deliriously happy?

HOW TO CREATE HAPPINESS

Menopause will force you to look at all areas of your life. You may start with the physical, dealing with hot flashes and weight gain, but if you don't look at the whole picture, you won't have the tools to achieve genuine happiness.

You can create happiness. Even out of great tragedy, the human spirit is capable of achieving happiness. Do you want to be happy? Believe it or not, it is *your* choice.

STEPS TO CREATING HAPPINESS

- Decide to be happy. Happiness is a choice.
- Relax and laugh more often. When you start to feel stressed, breathe deeply—try not to worry so much.
- Understand that happiness is not a full-time job.
- Find lessons in the challenges of life. What can you learn from a difficult situation? If you can take away a life lesson from a challenging situation, it is easier to get past negative feelings so you can be happy.

- Live in the present. You cannot fix the past and you do not know what the future holds. Embrace the now.
- Be grateful for the many gifts in your life.
- Accept yourself— remember the "perfect you" inside.
- Be a positive thinker.
- Create goals that bring you joy.
- Focus on the journey, not the payoff.
- Visualize your dreams.
- Nourish healthy relationships in your life.
- Spoil your body. Pamper yourself. Eat well and exercise.
- Give back to others.
- Avoid smoking, drugs or excessive alcohol.
- Journal.

> Respect your body—it is
> the path to your spirit.

One of the strongest tools for personal growth is journaling. It is a safe place for expression. The process of writing allows you to analyze and contemplate your life. It is also a wonderful tool to sort out thoughts and feelings. Journaling can offer you healing, the opportunity to solve problems, awaken your spirit and strengthen your inner voice. Recording your feelings can offer you a new perspective and help you achieve balance in your life.

Find a special notebook, diary or journal and select a writing pen just for journaling. You can journal when you first wake up or some people prefer to journal in the quiet hours before bedtime. Whether you choose to journal in the morning or evening, journal daily.

Answer these questions before starting your journal—your answers will be a great springboard for you to start journaling.

HAPPINESS JOURNALING EXERCISE

What is your definition of happiness?

What things made you happy in your past?

What makes you happy now?

What areas from the Happiness Questionnaire need focus to create happiness?

Set goals in areas that you can improve. List five new goals that will improve your life.

Every morning write in your journal what you will do to make yourself happy, and how you will make others happy. What will you do today to be happy?

Surround yourself with positive people.

MANIFEST HAPPINESS: KEEP YOUR LIFE SIMPLE

You need space and clarity to create happiness. Simplifying your life—from your home to your schedule—can help create that space in your life. If your home is cluttered, clean up your space. Clutter is like a self-imposed fat suit—stop hiding under a mess. Get to the root of your cluttered life. Are you messy because you are lazy—how can a lazy person grow? Are you living in clutter to hide your disappointment in life—you cannot overcome disappointment by hiding from the truth. Clutter is a symptom of something not working in your life. This manifestation may hold you back from happiness.

If your to-do list is jam-packed every day, focus on tasks that make your life better and make you feel happy. We all have to shop for food, pay bills and do laundry. Spread your life's duties throughout the week, so each day has free time scheduled for you. When you have the burden of chores or tasks weighing on your spirit, you cannot grow. It's like throwing a brick on a plant: It cannot grow and shine squashed under the brick. Lift the brick of too many chores or tasks that can be managed over time. Manage your life, honoring that you are the number-one priority. Sometimes you may have to say no—you don't have to do everything for everyone. Focus on you.

Simplify your life.

MAKEOVER TIPS

- Make time for yourself.
- Remember that you don't have to say "yes" to everything.
- Simplify your life.
- Delegate—you don't have to do everything yourself.
- Declutter your house.
- Have a good attitude.
- Set small, attainable goals.
- Reward your progress.
- Share your goals with loved ones, so you are accountable.

A GOOD ATTITUDE OPENS THE DOOR TO HAPPINESS

Have you noticed that cranky, crabby people are usually not happy people? No matter what your life situation, having a good attitude can open the door to your happiness. What exactly is a good attitude? It has to do with how you interpret your current situation. Being optimistic allows you to attract good situations and good people into your life. A good attitude can actually improve your stress levels and health. By practicing a hopeful outlook, you are telling yourself and the world that you believe good things will come your way. When you are negative, that pessimistic outlook can actually attract bad results. Usually, fear fuels negativity. If you start having a bad attitude, ask yourself, "What am I afraid of?" What is the underlying fear behind this negative attitude? Practice saying to yourself every day, "No matter what happens today, I will see the good."

> Positive Thoughts + Positive Action =
> Good Attitude

THE MENOPAUSE MAKEOVER
HAPPINESS PRESCRIPTION

- Empower yourself to embrace change.
- Accept change; it is the only constant in life.
- If you have the courage to change, happiness is your choice.

- Acknowledge your possibilities.
- Give thanks for what you have.
- Live in the present, so you can witness happiness.

HOW TO GET WHAT YOU WANT IN LIFE

After evaluating happiness in your life, you may be asking, "So what do I want in life and how do I get it?" As women, we often focus our attention on what other people want, and we try to make sure they get it. Often we have no idea what makes us happy, other than being with the people we love. Many women arrive at the menopause transition completely clueless as to what makes them happy or what they want out of life.

Examine areas in your life denying you personal fulfillment; the Happiness Questionnaire can give you a head start. Setting goals is one of the simplest, most effective ways to create change and navigate the path toward happiness. These journal exercises can be very motivating. Once you identify your goals, you will be able to track results (more on goal-setting in Chapter 12) to build self-confidence.

GOAL-SETTING EXERCISE

Forms for these goal-setting exercises can be found in Chapter 12 on page 321.

- List everything you have ever wanted to do in your lifetime. How can you start turning these dreams into realities?

- Make a list from the Happiness Question-naire, starting with the lowest score. Next to each area, jot down what you can do to add happi-ness to that area.

- Each week, go down that list and start incorporating an "action" you can do to improve these areas.

- Set short-term and long-term goals. Set daily, monthly, 6-month, 1-year and 5-year goals. Refer to your list daily. Visualize reaching your goals.

Once you begin seeing results, reward yourself. Celebrate. Creating a life you want to live is a powerful tool to living joyfully.

- Be clear and concise in your goal-setting. For example: I want to travel and see the world (a vague goal). A more concise goal: I want to see Italy, Spain and Greece by the end of next year (a focused, achievable goal). If money is an issue, set a goal to raise money or get a small weekend job—and start saving.

- Set realistic goals.
- Update your goals. When a new desire comes up, add it to the list.
- Prioritize your goals.
- Have small and large goals. You will reach some faster than others. Some may be complex and need more time.
- Every day, record your actions toward obtaining your goals.

GRATITUDE

Using the power of gratitude is one of the easiest ways to create happiness in your life. We often go through our busy days without acknowledging the wonderful gifts that surround us. Appreciating these blessings will create a positive attitude that will, in turn, attract happiness and abundance. People who are grateful often have better health and experience less stress. By practicing gratitude, you can increase your self-esteem and energy.

Often we resist events or people in our lives. This negative energy will assure only negative outcomes. Gratitude is a positive energy, attracting positive results. You will attract whatever energy you send out. It is easy to get caught up in being negative and angry when life does not go the way we want it. To break this destructive cycle, start examining your life and give thanks for all that is positive. Accept people or situations for what they are; this helps eliminate resistance in life. When you conquer resistance, you will attract happiness.

Acceptance + Gratitude = Happiness

GRATITUDE EXERCISE

○ Mentally make a list of all the things you feel grateful for. Sometimes you can find gratitude during prayer or a meditation session focused on thankfulness.

○ List 10 things you are grateful for:

1.

2.

3.

4.

5.

6.

7.

8.

9.

10.

- Let people know how special they are to you, and how thankful you are that they are in your life.
- When something negative happens, try to find the positive in it. Is there something to be thankful for in that experience?

MAKEOVER TAKE-ACTION LIST

- Reflect on your answers from the Happiness Questionnaire. In what areas can you increase your happiness? Set achievable goals for yourself.

- What steps do you need to take to create happiness? Refer to page 255.

- Complete the happiness journaling exercise on page 257.

- Declutter and simplify your life.

- Have a good attitude every day.

- Read the Menopause Makeover Happiness Formula once a week.

- Complete the goal-setting journaling exercise on pages 308-325.

- Complete the gratitude exercise on page 264.

- Discuss your goals with loved ones.

- Show appreciation for the people and things in your life.

- Be *happy!* You are about to begin your Menopause Makeover!

Happiness is a choice.

MAKEOVER TIPS

- Be aware and grateful for the good things in your life.
- Practice forgiveness.
- Focus your attention on happiness and positive thinking.

IN YOUR ESSENTIAL PLANNER

- Set happiness goals in your Month-at-a-Glance planner.
- Make a list of the things that make you happy and record them in your journal.
- Acknowledge people/things in your life daily in your 12-Week Planner.
- List things you are grateful for in your Gratitude List.
- Add a list of friends who you feel happy around to your Menopause Makeover Contacts.

PART TWO

Your Menopause Makeover:
Planning Your Transformation

chapter 10

Getting the Facts Straight: The 10 Facts You Need to Know to Be Successful

In Part Two, all the pieces of the puzzle come together to create the new you. You can personalize your Menopause Makeover in three easy steps.

1. Identify the facts and tools needed to begin your Makeover.
2. Create your health profile.
3. Set goals for your 12-week Makeover.

After completing these three steps, you are ready to begin the Menopause Makeover 12-Week Plan!

THE TEN MENOPAUSE MAKEOVER FACTS

Identify the facts and tools needed to begin your Makeover. To successfully set achievable goals, track your progress and stay motivated, you need to take stock of your current situation. In order to take 8 Menopause Makeover steps forward, you need to know where you stand.

THE TEN FACTS

FACT #1:	You have to get real to make changes
FACT #2:	The numbers don't lie: The BMI Chart
FACT #3:	You have an ideal weight unique only to you
FACT #4:	Knowing your proportions can save your life: The Waist-to-Hip Ratio
FACT #5:	Change is all about balance: Body fat and lean body mass
FACT #6:	Counting calories matters: What you put in your mouth can change your health
FACT #7:	Burning calories matters: The Basal Metabolic Rate (BMR)
FACT #8:	You gotta move to get anywhere! Exercise and physical activity can move you into a healthy future
FACT #9:	It takes energy to process food: The thermic effect of food
FACT #10:	You Must Commit to the Menopause Makeover Food Pyramid

FACT #1: YOU HAVE TO GET REAL TO MAKE CHANGES

Before you can set goals, you must get real with yourself. Whether you are addressing hot flashes or weight gain, or just trying to eat healthy and incorporate exercise in your daily routine, understanding your physical statistics will give you the opportunity to set attainable goals. Do you know your ideal weight? What percentage of your body weight is fat? How many calories do you need to maintain your current weight? What daily calorie intake will smooth the progress of achieving your perfect weight?

By getting real with yourself and facing the facts, you will increase your odds of accomplishing your Menopause Makeover goals successfully.

FACT #2: THE NUMBERS DON'T LIE: THE BMI CHART

One of the most common charts used for determining body fat is the BMI chart. *BMI* stands for "body mass index." The BMI calculation is a measurement of your body fat composition that uses a mathematical formula: your weight in kilograms, divided by your height in meters squared (BMI = kg/m2). Don't be intimidated by the math! The math has already been taken care of, so just check the BMI chart to easily get your body fat calculation. All you need to know is your height and current weight.

More than one third of adults in the United States are overweight or obese. Many health-care providers use the BMI chart as a gauge to monitor weight because it is inexpensive and easy to use. Being overweight can lead to serious health problems, such as heart disease, diabetes and cancer. In Chapter 11, I'll walk you through the process of determining your BMI. If your result is 18.5 to 24.9, you are within "normal" range. If your result is 25 to 29.9, you are overweight; 30 and above, you are obese.

The BMI chart is a great tool, but it does not account for your body composition. If you are muscle-bound (muscle weighs more than fat), your BMI chart results may categorize you as obese when, in fact, you are healthy. If you are over 50 years of age with a lesser amount of amount of muscle mass, the BMI chart may underestimate your weight. If you are muscle-bound or have a lesser amount of muscle mass and are over the age of 50, you may wish to use the lean body weight formula in Chapter 11 for a more accurate calculation.

FACT #3: YOU HAVE AN IDEAL WEIGHT UNIQUE ONLY TO YOU

Many skinny celebrities we see on television spend a lot of time maintaining those slender silhouettes. From my work as a producer, I know firsthand some of the challenges that celebrities experience while striving to maintain their girlish figures. A famous friend of mine is short and square in build. She will never have that tall, lean, skinny look. It is not her body type. Yet she is very healthy—she eats well, exercises daily and she looks great! She honors her ideal weight.

In Chapter 11 we will calculate your healthy weight, so you can begin accepting your perfect size. Do not be influenced by the media's interpretation of beauty. Everybody is different! Your frame, bone structure and body composition are unique to you.

FACT #4: KNOWING YOUR PROPORTIONS CAN SAVE YOUR LIFE: THE WAIST-TO-HIP RATIO

The BMI chart is a good weight gauge. Where we hold our fat—hips or belly—can indicate our health risks. Women with pear-shaped bodies, who carry their weight on the hips, have a lower risk of health issues, such as coronary heart disease, diabetes, blood pressure and obesity. Women who carry the majority of their weight around the middle, the "apple" body shape, have a higher risk of health concerns. A waist-to-hip ratio above 0.85 puts you at risk. For women with apple body shapes, it is important to keep excess fat off that midsection. This is a true challenge during menopause. My menopause fat was lumped in the middle, putting me in the unhealthy category! It took hard work to reduce that menopause midsection. You will measure your waist and hips to determine your waist-to-hip ratio in Chapter 11.

FACT #5: CHANGE IS ALL ABOUT BALANCE: BODY FAT AND LEAN BODY MASS

After you determine your BMI, we will calculate how much body fat and lean body mass (muscles, organs, bones) you have. This exercise will show you how much fat your body is carrying. During menopause, fat shifts to the midsection, so you will determine both your body fat and lean body mass in the next chapter. Remember, you can turn fat into muscle. After I initially calculated my lean body mass and body fat (a whopping 38 percent!), I became committed to a daily exercise routine. I was determined to turn that fat back into muscle! Knowing exactly how much fat and lean body mass you have will allow you to set goals you can track. Build muscle; it will burn fat! You will be stronger and feel better.

FACT #6: COUNTING CALORIES MATTERS: WHAT YOU PUT IN YOUR MOUTH CAN CHANGE YOUR HEALTH

A calorie is a unit of energy, a measurement. It is the amount of energy it takes to raise the temperature of 1 gram of water 1.8 degrees Fahrenheit. You can consume calories and burn calories. For many of us, a calorie is a pain in the butt—or a pound on our menopausal midsection. As discussed in Chapter 3, counting calories can change your health profile. As we age and lose muscle mass, we need fewer calories to survive. Knowing how many calories you need to consume in order to maintain, lose or add weight is an important step during the Menopause Makeover. Whether you are a vegetarian or a meat-lover, the number of calories you consume and burn each day will affect your health.

One pound of fat equals 3,500 calories. Consuming 500 fewer calories per day for one week equals one pound of fat. In the next chapter, you will calculate your current calorie consumption and calorie needs. Then you will use this number to manage your food intake and physical activity during the 12-Week Menopause Makeover. Using the food planner template in Chapter 13 will give you the tools to stay on track with your calorie goal.

FACT #7: BURNING CALORIES MATTERS: THE BASAL METABOLIC RATE (BMR)

The minimum calories needed to keep you alive (heartbeat, breathing) while you are asleep is called your Basal Metabolic Rate (BMR). It is the smallest amount of energy burned by the body in a resting state. Your BMR number can be used to calculate the speed of your metabolism—the rate your body burns calories—so you can determine how many calories you need to maintain, lose or increase your weight.

Both genetics and environment figure in your BMR. For example, some people are born with a high metabolism. Men have more muscle mass, so their metabolism is higher than a woman's. Your BMR goes down as you age. These are all factors you cannot change.

Your weight and body fat percentage both affect BMR. These factors *can* be changed. Exercise can raise your BMR; and exercise creates muscles, increasing BMR.

Your Basal Metabolic Rate is the largest factor (60–70 percent) in your total calorie expenditure. Calculating your BMR is the first part of the equation used in determining how many calories your body requires at its current weight. In the next chapter, you'll calculate your BMR to figure out your caloric needs for your Menopause Makeover.

FACT #8: YOU GOTTA MOVE TO GET ANYWHERE! EXERCISE AND PHYSICAL ACTIVITY CAN MOVE YOU INTO A HEALTHY FUTURE

The second factor in your total calorie expenditure (20–30%) is how much energy your body expends during physical activity. Refer to the Calories Burned Per Hour chart in Chapter 4 to calculate the energy you expend during physical activity. Consider adding a few new activities to your daily routine.

FACT #9: IT TAKES ENERGY TO PROCESS FOOD: THE THERMIC EFFECT OF FOOD

The third factor in your total calorie expenditure is the thermic effect of food. This refers to the amount of energy it takes your body to digest food. It takes your body more energy to process protein than fat, with carbohydrates falling in the middle. Why does this matter for your makeover? Knowing what foods speed up your metabolism can help you lose weight. Exercise can also speed up your metabolism, as discussed in Chapter 4. When you eat foods that can speed up your metabolism, combined with exercise, you have a winning formula. More good news: While you are sleeping, resting and eating, your body is also burning energy.

FACT #10: YOU MUST COMMIT TO THE MENOPAUSE MAKEOVER FOOD PYRAMID

It is important to fuel your body with the proper nutrients every day. Eating a properly balanced meal three times a day, along with two to three snacks, will ensure that your metabolism stays active, your body is nourished and you maintain a healthy weight for your Menopause Makeover. The Menopause Makeover Food Pyramid provides you with the correct proportions of calories from protein, carbohydrates and fats—exactly what your body needs to be healthy during menopause! See Chapter 3 for more information.

THE MENOPAUSE MAKEOVER FOOD PYRAMID

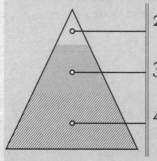

25% of calories from healthy fats

35% of calories from low-fat, lean protein

40% of calories from low- to medium-glycemic carbs

MAKEOVER TIPS

Don't skip the next chapter. Chapter 11 will help you craft your personal caloric needs and weight-loss goals. It is one of the most important chapters in this book! Without your starting numbers, you have no reference point for setting and tracking goals.

MAKEOVER TAKE-ACTION LIST

- Purchase a fabric tape measure to be used in Chapter 11.
- Make sure you have a calibrated scale.
- Make a copy of the Menopause Makeover Food Pyramid located on page 92 and tape it to your refrigerator.

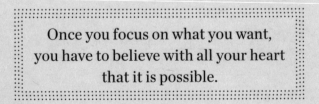

Once you focus on what you want, you have to believe with all your heart that it is possible.

chapter 11

Putting It All Together:
Doing the Math Is an Equation
for Success

As my waistline was rapidly expanding, I finally had to admit that my health and beauty were quickly declining. Menopause had become a runaway train, and I was tied to the tracks of my youthful past.

When I created the Menopause Makeover, I decided to take a "before" photograph in my favorite swimsuit and take measurements, so I would have a reference point to set goals. I was too embarrassed to ask my husband to take the "before" photograph, for fear that he would regret marrying me, so I secretly packed my swimsuit, grabbed a tripod along with the family digital camera and took a self-portrait body shot in my office. What happened next shook my world. When I downloaded my bikini pictures, I was horrified—I was fat! My favorite swimsuit was stretched over my hips as if I had squeezed into a child's swimsuit. Sobbing as if someone had died, I feared I would never return to my healthy, sexy self again. To add salt to the wound, as I was downing a chocolate-covered donut I took out the tape measure and documented my sorry statistics.

An hour passed of feeling hopeless, old and ugly, staring at this new depressing evidence. Then something interesting happened. Knowing the awful truth was actually liberating. There was no more avoiding the hard fact that going through menopause completely changed my body shape, skin, moods and outlook on life—and not for the better. I asked myself, "Do I give up and let this transition get the better of me, or do I arm myself with information and take action?"

After I reviewed my statistics and looked at the hideous photograph, I decided I needed some inspiration. I found a photograph of a healthy me taken a few years earlier for inspiration (you can see those photographs in the Introduction). Next I did some calculations so I knew what healthy was for my size, then set attainable goals. Those terrifying measurements actually kicked me in the butt to make changes.

In this chapter you will do some math—don't worry, the formulas are easy!—to take stock of your current health profile and determine your personal makeover goals. You will record your statistics and find a photograph taken of you in the past when you felt good about yourself to use as inspiration for your makeover.

You may feel resistance to this part of your Menopause Makeover. Who among us is friends with a tape measure and likes math? But it is this part of your makeover that will reflect the truth about your health profile. Understanding your personal statistics will allow you to face your demons. Once you set goals that can change your health, your demons will crumble under the sword of knowledge. You will have power over your life again. Doing the math is an equation for success!

CREATE YOUR HEALTH PROFILE

This chapter is the second step needed to begin your Menopause Makeover. It includes all the calculations you will use when you create your personal Menopause Makeover in the Essential Planner. You'll refer to this chapter throughout the 12-Week Plan.

CALCULATE YOUR BODY MASS INDEX

Calculate your body mass index using the BMI chart on the next page.

Locate your height at the top of this chart and your weight on the left side. Determine your current body mass index.

MY **BMI** IS > _____

BODY MASS INDEX (BMI) CHART

BMI	Height (in)								
	58	59	60	61	62	63	64	65	66
Wgt. (lbs)	4'10"	4'11"	5'0"	5'1"	5'2"	5'3"	5'4"	5'5"	5'6"
100	21	20	20	19	18	18	17	17	16
105	22	21	21	20	19	19	18	18	17
110	23	22	22	21	20	20	19	18	18
115	24	23	23	22	21	20	20	19	19
120	25	24	23	23	22	21	21	20	19
125	26	25	24	24	23	22	22	21	20
130	27	26	25	25	24	23	22	22	21
135	28	27	26	26	25	24	23	23	22
140	29	28	27	27	26	25	24	23	23
145	30	29	28	27	27	26	25	24	23
150	31	30	29	28	27	27	26	25	24
155	32	31	30	29	28	28	27	26	25
160	34	32	31	30	29	28	28	27	26
165	35	33	32	31	30	29	28	28	27
170	36	34	33	32	31	30	29	28	27
175	37	35	34	33	32	31	30	29	28
180	38	36	35	34	33	32	31	30	29
185	39	37	36	35	34	33	32	31	30
190	40	38	37	36	35	34	33	32	31
195	41	39	38	37	36	35	34	33	32
200	42	40	39	38	37	36	34	33	32
205	43	41	40	39	38	36	35	34	33
210	44	43	41	40	38	37	36	35	34
215	45	44	42	41	39	38	37	36	35
220	46	45	43	42	40	39	38	37	36
225	47	46	44	43	41	40	39	38	36
230	48	47	45	44	42	41	40	38	37
235	49	48	46	44	43	42	40	39	38
240	50	49	47	45	44	43	41	40	39
245	51	50	48	46	45	43	42	41	40
250	52	51	49	47	46	44	43	42	40
255	53	52	50	48	47	45	44	43	41
260	54	53	51	49	48	46	45	43	42
265	56	54	52	50	49	47	46	44	43
270	57	55	53	51	49	48	46	45	44
275	58	56	54	52	50	49			

BODY MASS INDEX (BMI) CHART

67	68	69	70	71	72	73	74	75	76
5'7"	5'8"	5'9"	5'10"	5'11"	6'0"	6'1"	6'2"	6'3"	6'4"
16	15	15	14	14	14	13	13	13	12
16	16	16	15	15	14	14	14	13	13
17	17	16	16	15	15	15	14	14	13
18	18	17	17	16	16	15	15	14	14
19	18	18	17	17	16	16	15	15	15
20	19	18	18	17	17	17	16	16	15
20	20	19	19	18	18	17	17	16	16
21	21	20	19	19	18	18	17	17	16
22	21	21	20	20	19	19	18	18	17
23	22	21	21	20	20	19	19	18	18
24	23	22	22	21	20	20	19	19	18
24	24	23	22	22	21	20	20	19	19
25	24	24	23	22	22	21	21	20	20
26	25	24	24	23	22	22	21	21	20
27	26	25	24	24	23	22	22	21	21
27	27	26	25	24	24	23	23	22	21
28	27	27	26	25	24	24	23	23	22
29	28	27	27	26	25	24	24	23	23
30	29	28	27	27	26	25	24	24	23
31	30	29	28	27	27	26	25	24	24
31	30	30	29	28	27	26	26	25	24
32	31	30	29	29	28	27	26	26	25
33	32	31	30	29	29	28	27	26	26
34	33	32	31	30	29	28	28	27	26
35	34	33	32	31	30	29	28	28	27
35	34	33	32	31	31	30	29	28	27
36	35	34	33	32	31	30	30	29	28
37	36	35	34	33	32	31	30	29	29
38	37	36	35	34	33	32	31	30	29
38	37	36	35	34	33	32	32	31	30
39	38	37	36	35	34	33	32	31	30
40	39	38	37	36	35	34	33	32	31
41	40	38	37	36	35	34	33	33	32
42	40	39	38	37	36	35	34	33	32
42	41	40	39	38	37	36	35	34	33

BMI CATEGORIES

- Underweight = <18.5
- Normal weight = 18.5–24.9
- Overweight = 25–29.9
- Obese = BMI of 30 or greater

Record your BMI in "Statistics: For Your Eyes Only" on page 301 in this chapter under the Current Statistics column. Your BMI number will be one gauge used to monitor your health throughout the Menopause Makeover.

CALCULATE YOUR IDEAL WEIGHT

No two bodies are alike. The combination of your body type, frame size and body composition will determine your ideal weight.

Go back to the BMI chart and look at the weights for your height in the "normal" category (18.5–24.9). This will give you a healthy range to strive for.

EXAMPLE > 5'6" woman would have a normal weight range within 110 and 155 pounds.

EXAMPLE > 5'7" woman would have a normal weight range between 115 to 160 pounds.

Understanding your health risks will help you set goals and track results.

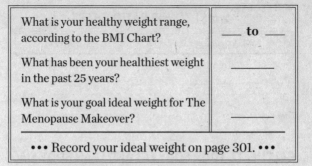

What is your healthy weight range, according to the BMI Chart?	____ to ____
What has been your healthiest weight in the past 25 years?	_____
What is your goal ideal weight for The Menopause Makeover?	_____

••• Record your ideal weight on page 301. •••

CALCULATE YOUR WAIST-TO-HIP RATIO

To determine whether you have a healthy waist-to-hip ratio, use a fabric measuring tape and measure the circumference of your hips at the widest part of your buttocks. Then measure your waist at the smallest circumference of your natural waist, usually just above the belly button.

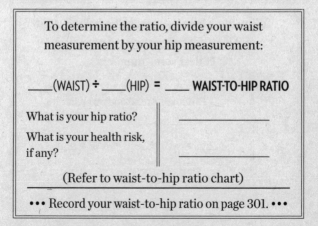

To determine the ratio, divide your waist measurement by your hip measurement:

____(WAIST) ÷ ____(HIP) = ____ **WAIST-TO-HIP RATIO**

What is your hip ratio? _____

What is your health risk, if any? _____

(Refer to waist-to-hip ratio chart)

••• Record your waist-to-hip ratio on page 301. •••

WAIST-TO-HIP RATIO CHART

Measurement	Health Risk
0.80 or below	Low
0.81–0.85	Moderate
0.85+	High

CALCULATE YOUR BODY FAT AND LEAN BODY MASS

Using the BMI chart gives you a healthy weight estimate based on height and weight. Next, we will calculate how many pounds of body fat and how many pounds of lean body mass (muscles, organs, bones) you are carrying, as well as your body fat percentage. These are excellent measurements to use to set goals for your Menopause Makeover.

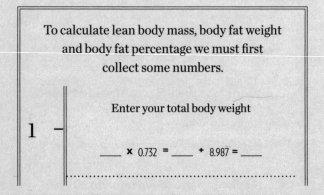

To calculate lean body mass, body fat weight and body fat percentage we must first collect some numbers.

1 —

Enter your total body weight

_____ × 0.732 = _____ + 8.987 = _____

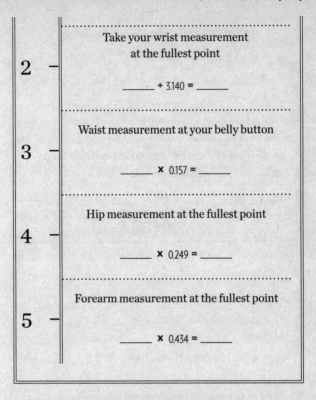

2 —
Take your wrist measurement
at the fullest point

_____ ÷ 3.140 = _____

3 —
Waist measurement at your belly button

_____ ✕ 0.157 = _____

4 —
Hip measurement at the fullest point

_____ ✕ 0.249 = _____

5 —
Forearm measurement at the fullest point

_____ ✕ 0.434 = _____

Once you calculate #1 through #5, use these numbers
for the next three formulas.

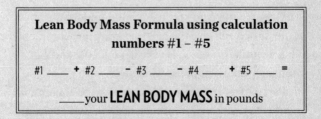

**Lean Body Mass Formula using calculation
numbers #1 – #5**

#1 ____ **+** #2 ____ **–** #3 ____ **–** #4 ____ **+** #5 ____ **=**

____your **LEAN BODY MASS** in pounds

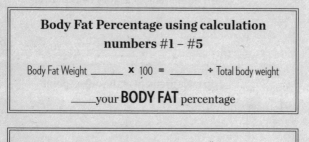

Body Fat Weight Formula using calculation numbers #1 – #5

Total body weight _____ – Lean Body Mass _____ =

_____your **BODY FAT** in pounds

Body Fat Percentage using calculation numbers #1 – #5

Body Fat Weight _____ **×** 100 = _____ ÷ Total body weight

_____your **BODY FAT** percentage

How many pounds of lean body mass are you carrying?	_____
How many pounds of fat are you carrying?	_____
What is your body fat percentage?	_____

••• Go to page 301 and record your current lean body mass in pounds, body fat in pounds and body fat percentage. •••

Having your body fat calculated underwater by a professional will give the most accurate measurement. This formula, however, is very dependable and can be used for your Menopause Makeover.

Part of the Menopause Makeover exercise commitment is to turn that fat into muscle. This will increase your metabolism and decrease your risk of health concerns. As you start to tone up and feel better about your body, you will also get stronger—to "kick some butt" in other areas of your life.

CALCULATE YOUR CALORIE NEEDS AND SET CALORIE GOALS

This next section is dedicated to counting calories—how many you currently consume, and what you need to consume in order to achieve your perfect weight. If you honor these numbers, you will see results. The numbers don't lie!

First, calculate your Basal Metabolic Rate (BMR), the energy you are currently expending during physical activity, and the thermic effect of food to determine how many calories you need to maintain your current weight.

ACTUAL CALORIES YOU BURN

Calculate how many calories your body needs to maintain its current weight.

BMR **+** Energy Expended **+** Thermic Effect of Food **=**
CURRENT CALORIES YOUR BODY BURNS TODAY

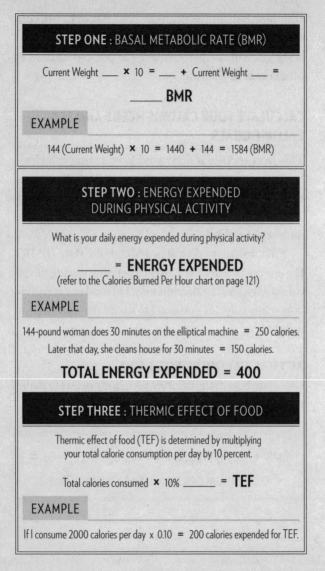

STEP ONE : BASAL METABOLIC RATE (BMR)

Current Weight ___ × 10 = ___ + Current Weight ___ =

_____ **BMR**

EXAMPLE

144 (Current Weight) × 10 = 1440 + 144 = 1584 (BMR)

STEP TWO : ENERGY EXPENDED DURING PHYSICAL ACTIVITY

What is your daily energy expended during physical activity?

_____ = **ENERGY EXPENDED**
(refer to the Calories Burned Per Hour chart on page 121)

EXAMPLE

144-pound woman does 30 minutes on the elliptical machine = 250 calories.

Later that day, she cleans house for 30 minutes = 150 calories.

TOTAL ENERGY EXPENDED = 400

STEP THREE : THERMIC EFFECT OF FOOD

Thermic effect of food (TEF) is determined by multiplying your total calorie consumption per day by 10 percent.

Total calories consumed × 10% _____ = **TEF**

EXAMPLE

If I consume 2000 calories per day x 0.10 = 200 calories expended for TEF.

CALCULATING CALORIES

An easy way to figure out how many calories you consume per day is to keep a food diary for seven days, counting every calorie. On the seventh day add up all your daily calorie totals and divide by seven days, giving you an average daily calorie consumption number. This strategy will give you a good average of how many total calories you are consuming daily.

STEP FOUR : TAKE THE PREVIOUS 3 CALCULATIONS AND APPLY

BMR _____ + Energy Expended _____ + TEF _____ =

_____ total calories used by the body to maintain your current weight.

EXAMPLE

1584 + 400 + 200 = 2184 calories required to maintain 144 pounds.

How many calories is your body currently burning to maintain its current weight?

_____

••• Record this number on page 301 under the "current" statistics column. •••

HOW MANY CALORIES DO YOU NEED TO CONSUME TO LOSE WEIGHT?

To lose one pound, you need to cut back 3,500 calories.

If you want to lose:

o ½ pound per week, subtract 250 food calories per day.
o 1 pound per week, subtract 500 food calories per day.
o 1½ pounds per week, subtract 750 food calories per day.
o 2 pounds per week, subtract 1,000 food calories per day.
o Taking exercise into account: ½ pound per week, eat 125 fewer calories and move 125 calories (a leisurely 30-minute walk).
o 1 pound per week, eat 250 fewer calories, move 250 more calories (a brisk 30-minute walk).
o 1½ pounds per week, eat 375 fewer calories, move 375 calories more.
o 2 pounds per week, 500 fewer calories of food per day, 500 calories more activity (take a brisk walk and vacuum the house like a madwoman).

CALCULATE YOUR CALORIE GOAL

There are two numbers you need in order to figure out your calorie goals. First you need to calculate how many calories you need to *cut* from your diet in order to lose weight. Using this number, you can figure out how many calories you should eat every day.

HOW MANY CALORIES SHOULD YOU CUT?

First, how many pounds per week do you want to lose?
____ Multiply this number by 3,500 to get the number

of calories you'd need to cut in one week to achieve this goal. To determine how many calories a day you'd need to cut in order to make this happen, divide the total calories by seven.

Losing one to two pounds per week is a healthy goal. If you have more than ten to fifteen pounds to lose, you may lose more than two pounds the first few weeks. Be realistic when setting your weight-loss goals. If you have 60 pounds to lose, plan on losing two pounds per week. That would take 30 weeks to meet your goal. The good news is you can use your 12-week Menopause Makeover Plan over and over until you achieve your goals.

EXAMPLE

If I want to lose 1 pound per week:
$1 \times 3{,}500 = 3{,}500$ fewer calories per week,
or 500 fewer calories per day.

HOW MANY CALORIES SHOULD YOU EAT PER DAY?

Now all you have to do is subtract the number of calories you should cut from the total number of calories you need per day to maintain your weight. Keep in mind that you should never consume fewer than 1,200 calories a day, or you risk putting your body into survival mode and *holding on* to calories instead of losing them!

EXAMPLE 1

I consume 2,184 calories per day and want to
lose 1 pound per week.
2,184 calories − 500 calories = 1,684 calories
per day to lose 1 pound per week.

EXAMPLE 2

I consume 2,184 calories per day and want to
lose 2 pounds per week.
2,184 calories − 1,000 calories = 1,184 calories
My adjusted goal would be 1,200 calories per
day to lose up to two pounds per week.

I decide to be less aggressive and lose 1 pound per
week. My plan is to cut 250 calories a day through exercise, and eat 250 fewer calories to cut a total of 500
calories a day. That is a plan I can live with. When you
create your plan, keep in mind your lifestyle and set
reasonable goals for yourself. (You can find these calculations online at www.menopausemakeover.com.)

Record your calorie-cutting goals on page 301 under
the "12-Week Goal" column.

Visualize the new you.

VISUALIZE THE POSSIBILITIES

After you collect current information and set your goals, the next step is to visualize your possibilities. If you have to lose 50 pounds to be healthy, set goals you can live with. Try losing one pound a week. Next year at this time, you will be at that healthy weight. It probably took years to gain that weight. Set realistic goals for yourself.

I gained 25 pounds in a very short period. I set an aggressive goal—two pounds per week. In 12 weeks I actually lost 25 pounds. I have managed to keep off 20 pounds of that consistently, and fluctuate 5 pounds, depending on holidays and travel. This is normal. I continue to practice my new healthy lifestyle by exercising five to six days a week and eating within my healthy calorie range. If I find myself gaining again, I go back on the plan to keep my weight under control.

I always feel better knowing that my health is above average. It is all a balancing act. The numbers don't lie! I am still shocked to look back at my previous numbers. It feels great to have accomplished my goals. Numbers held the key to my future—and they hold the key to yours, too.

Now that you know your numbers,
use them and believe with all your heart
that you deserve to be healthy.

STATISTICS: FOR YOUR EYES ONLY

Pull out that measuring tape; it's time to record your statistics. This may be the most depressing section of the Makeover. It was for me. Once I started my Menopause Makeover, these statistics were scary, yet liberating. Do not share this section with anyone. It is for your eyes only.

Why do we have to torture ourselves with this horrifying exercise? Because measuring yourself—seeing it in writing—may just be the kick in the pants you need to allow you to move forward.

For years, I thought my butt was the same size it was a decade ago. *Wrong.* It was four inches bigger. My waistline had grown *six* inches thicker! After a well-needed sob session, sitting naked in the bathroom with the tape measure, I got inspired. I picked up that photograph of myself taken a few years earlier, when I felt and looked good, and taped it to my bathroom mirror. I made copies of the photo and carried one around in my daily planner. I also taped a copy in my Menopause Makeover Planner. I looked at the photo every day. Twelve weeks later, I once again looked like the happy girl in that picture. Once you go through menopause, that waistline needs some extra attention. After the 12-Week Plan, I got my waistline back, and my health. It was a good pinch thicker than the old days, but at least it was an hourglass again . . . not a basketball.

MAKEOVER TIPS

I

- Be honest when calculating your "numbers."
- Use these calculations to track your performance.
- If you need help measuring yourself, ask a friend or a loved one.

DOCUMENT YOUR STATISTICS

Drag yourself into the bathroom. Strip down. Pull out that tape measure and start recording the hard truth, *your current statistics,* on page 301. Next, set realistic goals under the "12-Week Goal" column. After your Menopause Makeover, come back to this page and record your results. In just twelve weeks you can be on your way to a healthier you! These statistics will help you stay motivated, and allow you to track your goals. Find a photograph of a healthy you, after the age of 25 years old, to use as inspiration. Tape your inspirational photo on page 302.

MAKEOVER TIPS

- Use a soft, fabric tape measure. It may be easier to have someone help you take your measurements while you're standing.

- Make sure your scale is on level ground. Stand on the scale first thing in the morning, naked if possible. Good calibration is important.

- Measure your bust wearing a bra, if you normally wear one.

- Measure your abdomen just under your belly button.

- Measure your calf at the maximum circumference.

- Measure your thigh at the crotch level below the fold of your buns.

- Use the BMI chart to determine your correct body mass index.

- Wear the same clothes, or your birthday suit, when you measure again twelve weeks later.

- Pull the tape measure tight enough to stay in position, but not too tight.

- If you have blood pressure concerns, buy a blood pressure "cuff" to monitor your blood pressure. These can be purchased at most pharmacies.

- If you have cholesterol concerns, record the levels that you obtained from your health-care provider.

- Set realistic goals. Measurable results usually take four or more weeks.

MAKEOVER TIPS

○ Take a previous photograph of yourself and tape it on page 302, "Inspirational Me." Then record the date. Twelve weeks later, place your current photograph on the next page under "New Me."

STATISTICS: For Your Eyes Only

Start Date _____   End Date _____

		CURRENT	12-WEEK GOAL	RESULTS
Height				
Neck				
Upper arms				
Bust				
Waist				
Abdomen				
Hips				
Waist-to-Hip Ratio				
Thighs				
BMI				
Lean body mass				
Body fat (lbs)				
Body fat (%)				
Calves				
Calories to maintain	Calories to lose			
Blood pressure				
Cholesterol				
Weight	Ideal Weight			

INSPIRATIONAL ME PHOTO

Date:

NEW ME PHOTO

Date:

MAKEOVER TAKE-ACTION LIST

- Do all the calculations in this chapter.
- Record these numbers in the appropriate places in the Menopause Makeover.

IN YOUR ESSENTIAL PLANNER

- Use your new calorie intake goal in the 12-Week Planner.
- Subtract exercise and activity calories from food intake calories to record your total daily calorie intake in the 12-Week Planner.
- Track your results using your Weekly Progress Report.

chapter 12

Setting Goals:
If You Write It Down, You Can
Make It Happen

After reading Part One, you are armed with knowledge. After doing the personal calculations, you are empowered with truth. Knowledge combined with truth is a winning formula for setting goals.

SET GOALS FOR YOUR 12-WEEK MAKEOVER

Setting goals will allow you to track successes and challenges. This is your personalized portion of the Menopause Makeover.

For some unexplained reason, I have set annual goals since I was 12 years old. In those early years, my goals were simple: Get straight A's on my report card; practice the piano; learn how to sew so I could make a pair of hot pants (my mom would not let me buy them); keep out of trouble; protect my brother and his hamster; play Little Kiddles with my friends. I witnessed at an early age that if I made a list of goals inspired by my dreams, they almost always miraculously happened. Goal-setting works, no matter what your age.

Now my goals are larger, encompassing more areas of my life. Every year on New Year's Day, I sit down and write goals. I include long- and short-term goals. I have personal goals, and goals for my relationship. Each year I save these goals. I love to look back and see the power of realized goals. My life is richer in all areas, thanks to goal-setting.

The process of asking what you want or need to be happy is a powerful exercise. This is often difficult for women. We are committed to others—often forgetting, or not even knowing, what we need to make ourselves happy. Goal-setting can change your life, whether you need to manage menopause symptoms, revamp your image, create or re-create a stimulating career, or work on a more intimate relationship.

In earlier chapters you were asked to fill out portions of this section, so you have already started. Take some quiet time and reflect on your goals. Be honest, dig deep and dream big!

MAKEOVER TIPS

- Identify what you want.
- Write it down.
- Be committed to taking the action needed to make it happen.
- Believe in yourself.
- Believe that your goals are possible.
- Tap into your dreams.
- When you have quiet time, visualize achieving your goals. What will your life look like? How will you feel?
- Be grateful for goals realized.
- Be grateful for lessons learned from unrealized goals.
- Be excited about your life embracing these new goals; this energy creates results.
- Be an inspiration to yourself and others.

MAKEOVER TAKE-ACTION LIST

- Review your goals weekly.
- Add new goals.
- Share your goals with others—being accountable to others can yield faster results.

IN YOUR ESSENTIAL PLANNER

- ○ Record all actions to achieve your goals in your Month-at-a-Glance Planner.
- ○ Write about your goals in your journal.

YOUR PERSONAL GOALS

Start Date :............:   End Date :............:

OVERALL MENOPAUSE MAKEOVER GOAL

:...:
:   :
:   :
:   :
:...:

What is your action plan to achieve this goal?

:...:
:   :
:   :
:...:

HORMONES

How will you address menopause symptoms?

What health concerns need attention?

What action will you take to manage these health concerns?

NUTRITION

What are your nutrition goals?

How will you achieve these goals?

How will you achieve these goals?

What are your big "food challenges"?

How will you conquer these challenges?

What supplements have you chosen for the
12-Week Plan?

What is your daily calorie intake to achieve or maintain a healthy weight?

How will you achieve this?

EXERCISE

What daily exercise activities have you chosen for the 12-Week Plan?

How long will you do these exercises each day?

How many days per week?

What is your target heart rate?

What was your health rating result from the
One-Mile Walk Fitness Test (page 135)?

How will you improve this rating?

If you dread exercising, how will you overcome this
attitude?

BEAUTY

What are your overall beauty goals?

How will you achieve them?

What are your goals for:
1. Your skin-care regimen

2. Your hairstyle/color

3. Your wardrobe

What age-embracing tips will you practice (refer to pages 147 to 149)?

What makeup tips will you incorporate (refer to page 171)?

What styling tips will you incorporate (refer to page 178)?

EMOTIONS

What areas of your emotional life need a Makeover?

How will you address:

1. Crankiness

2. Moodiness

3. Depression

4. Memory loss/fuzzy thinking

5. Stress

RELATIONSHIPS

What is the most important goal regarding your primary love relationship?

What relationships need extra attention?
1. Family

2. Friends

3. Coworkers

4. Neighbors

5. Others

How will you address these relationship challenges?

SPIRITUALITY AND HAPPINESS

How will you nurture your spirit?

How will you nurture your passions and fulfill your purpose in life?

How will you make a difference in your life?

How will you create happiness in your life?

Review all areas of happiness (page 253).
What are your short-term happiness goals?

What are your long-term happiness goals?

What dreams do you want to manifest in your lifetime?

How can you achieve them?

How can you simplify your life?

In which areas of your life do you need to practice forgiveness?

When you successfully complete *The Menopause Makeover,* how will you reward yourself?

LIVING YOUR DREAMS

List your dreams:

How can you start making these dreams realities?

From the Happiness Questionnaire (page 253),
what areas can you improve?

What is your action plan?

ACTION PLAN

Areas that need to be addressed:
Health

Love (with someone special)

Spirituality

Self-esteem

Work

Money (Do you feel safe?)

Hobbies

Friends

Relatives

Children

Home

Travel/adventure

Education/learning

Neighborhood

Giving

Creativity

Each week review this list and start incorporating an "action" to promote improvement. Set short-term goals (1 month, 3 months and 6 months):

Set long-term goals (1 year and 5 years):

Refer to your list daily. Visualize goals being achieved. Update your goals. When a new desire comes up, add it to the list. Create positive goals. Prioritize your goals. Set small and large goals. Some will be achieved faster than others. Some may be complex and need time. Set realistic goals.

Every day, record in your Essential Planner the actions needed to achieve your goals.

TAKING THE VOW: SAYING "I DO" TO THE NEW YOU

The Menopause Makeover embraces celebration! You have taken the steps to personalize your Menopause Makeover, and set your goals. It is time to say "I do" to the new you! Just like marriage, taking a vow (a solemn promise to perform a certain act) can be a fun way to verbalize your Menopause Makeover commitment to yourself and the people you love. Giving yourself a party to launch your Menopause Makeover celebrates your commitment to the journey you are about to begin. Selecting an attractive reward for accomplishing your goals is a great incentive to stay on course.

Your Menopause Makeover can take as much effort as planning a wedding. Why not incorporate some of the fun stuff weddings include? Planning a party with your close friends and family is a fantastic way to show the world that you are serious about your Menopause Makeover commitment. Perhaps your friends are struggling with menopause as well. Invite them to join you in the Menopause Makeover—you can all celebrate the start of your journey together!

CELEBRATE THE NEW YOU

Personalize your Menopause Makeover with a party theme unique to you. Are you an earthy-type person? If so, plan an "Overnight Backyard Camping Party" with a few good girlfriends. Are you a diva? Perhaps the "Diva Party" will be the perfect fit for you. Customize your party, and celebrate *you*. Here are a few ideas to get you started:

Afternoon tea party
Invite friends to enjoy "afternoon tea" Saturday or Sunday between 3 and 5 p.m.

Margarita hot-flash fiesta
Dust off the blender and whip up some yummy margaritas. Announce when you have a hot flash, and all the guests have to take a sip of their margarita.

Spa party
Book manicures and pedicures at your local salon or spa. Invite your girlfriends to an afternoon of pampering dedicated to your Menopause Makeover. Or book a manicurist and pedicurist to come to your home for an evening of luxury. If you really want to go all-out, book one of the many resort spas that host spa parties for groups. Make your Menopause Makeover an event!

Makeover and a meal
This is always a crowd-pleaser. Book a makeup artist and invite your girlfriends over for dinner. As you enjoy the evening with good friends, everyone gets a personalized makeup makeover. Take before and after photos. Often a Mary Kay™ or Avon™ representative can provide products and consultation for the group as you party.

Diva party

Embrace your inner diva with a Diva dinner party. Everyone must dress as a diva. Hire your own paparazzi.

THE RING: YOUR COMMITMENT TO YOURSELF

Before you take the Menopause Makeover vow, select a ring that you will wear on your right hand for the next 12 weeks. I located my grandmother's wedding ring. I had it sized and polished. As I wear her ring on my right-hand ring finger, I am inspired by her memory. You may have a college ring that holds good memories. Perhaps you want to purchase a new ring for this occasion. Or maybe someone special in your life would like to give you a ring to honor your Menopause Makeover.

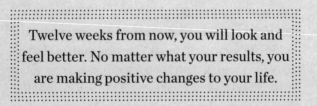

Twelve weeks from now, you will look and feel better. No matter what your results, you are making positive changes to your life.

Next, take the Menopause Makeover vow. You can read this vow privately to yourself or in front of loved ones.

THE MENOPAUSE MAKEOVER VOW

I promise to accept responsibility for my health.

I promise to love my natural beauty.

I promise to work hard at achieving my goals.

I promise to have an open mind to what is possible.

I promise to take action to achieve positive change.

I promise to nourish my body with healthy food.

I promise to exercise and stay active.

I promise to seek support when I need it.

I promise to forgive those who have hurt me.

I promise to be grateful for my blessings.

I promise to celebrate my spirit every day.

I promise to encourage others.

I promise to manifest good things for myself.

I promise to live in the present moment.

I promise to love myself in sickness and in health, for richer or poorer, forevermore.

After you take the Menopause Makeover vow, slip that special ring on your right ring finger. You just made a big commitment to your health, beauty and life.

THE MENOPAUSE MAKEOVER REWARD

Congratulations! You have made an important vow to change your life. Select a reward to enjoy when you complete your Menopause Makeover. It can be inexpensive, or expensive. It should be something special to you. You are about to begin 12 weeks of life-changing action. There will be struggles, challenges and frustrations—along with big successes. All of life's transitions are interwoven with ups and downs. Having a reward at the end of this journey can be a great motivator. My initial reward was fitting into the beautiful wedding gown my mother had given me for my special day! The next time I did the 12-Week Plan, my reward was a new wardrobe for my new body. My husband went shopping with me and helped pick out some flattering, sexy outfits.

Your Menopause Makeover journey will also provide rewards you cannot buy. Treat yourself when you complete the Menopause Makeover.

Now it's time to begin *your* Menopause Makeover!

MAKEOVER TIPS

- Select a party theme that is personal to you. Be proud to celebrate your new beginning. If you are happy about it, everyone will be happy for you.

- Get excited about the next 12 weeks—have fun!

- Take your vow seriously.

- Wear your ring joyfully. The Menopause Makeover is about a commitment to you.

IN YOUR ESSENTIAL PLANNER

- Tape a picture of your reward on your Menopause Makeover Reward page.

- Schedule your Menopause Makeover party in your Month-at-a-Glance Planner.

- Track results in your Weekly Progress Report.

PART THREE

Your Menopause Makeover
Essential Planner:
12 Weeks to a New You

chapter 13

The Essential Planner: Charting Your Success

So now you are informed, you've done your calculations and set goals, and you made a commitment to your Menopause Makeover. This section provides the tools you need to chart your success. If you write it down, you can create it, be it, do it and achieve it.

THE MENOPAUSE MAKEOVER TOOLS

- **Month-at-a-Glance Planner:** Use this calendar to keep track of your appointments.

- **Your Menopause Makeover Contacts:** Record contact information for your support group and Makeover Contacts.

- **Medical Forms:** Prepare your medical forms from Chapter 1 for your next doctor's appointment, and review the medical tests for your age group.

- **Menopause Makeover Food Plan:** Prepare your food plan every week to stay on track with your nutrition goals.

- **Menopause Makeover Shopping List:** Use the shopping list to ensure that your cart is loaded with healthy food.

- **Menopause Makeover Daily Meal Diary:** Make a habit of using this daily. It is one of the most important tools for your makeover.

- **Your 12-Week Plan:** Document medications, hormones and exercise daily.

- **Weekly Progress Report:** Chart your progress with this weekly report.

- **Your Gratitude List:** Record the things/people for which/whom you are grateful.

- **Your Menopause Makeover Reward:** Stay motivated with this reminder of how you'll reward yourself when you achieve your goals.

- **Journal Pages:** Keep a journal of your feelings.

- **Notes:** If you have an idea, question or need a reminder, jot it down.

All these tools will help you stay on track for a successful makeover. While you can write in these actual pages, you may want to use them as a template to create your own Menopause Makeover binder—you can copy the Month-at-a-Glance Planner, the Food Plan, the Shopping List, the Daily Meal Diary, the 12-Week Plan and the Weekly Progress Report so that you will have enough to use for all 12 weeks of the Makeover. Or you can download these forms from my Web site at www.menopausemakeover.com.

This chapter is dedicated to making your dreams come true!

MONTH-AT-A-GLANCE PLANNER

Doctor's visits, exercise dates, new beauty regimens, shopping dates, lunch with supportive friends, meetings with your spiritual group and dates with your loved ones—there's so much to keep track of!

Use this monthly planner to keep track of all your appointments, and witness your transformation during the *12-Week Menopause Makeover!*

MONTH:

SUN	MON	TUE	WED	THUR	FRI	SAT

MAKEOVER TIPS

1	Record all activities and appointments for your 12-Week Menopause Makeover on the Month-at-a-Glance Planner.
2	"Starting weight" is your original weight when you start the 12-Week Plan.
3	Track your menopause symptoms. Use the chart on page 15.
4	Be honest about your emotions.
5	Set goals in the exercise section. For example, are you just trying to include exercise in your life? Or are you trying to increase intensity and duration for better results? Push yourself—you will be amazed at the outcome. If you get bored, ask a friend to join you or change your activity.
6	Purchase a heart-rate monitor watch, if you don't use exercise equipment with this information. Your heart rate will allow you to track and monitor your intensity. This is a great tool to use when exercising and setting goals.
7	You can use the Calories Burned Per Hour chart on page 121 to calculate calories in "other activity."
8	If you wake up and eat at 6 a.m., make sure you have a midmorning snack. If you eat breakfast at 8–9 a.m., do not add a midmorning snack.
9	Calculating calories is one of the most important tasks you can do in this journal entry. After the first couple of weeks it will become easier, because you will know the calorie information for your favorite foods. Stick with it and it will pay off.
10	Be honest with yourself regarding the areas that need work. Acknowledging challenges is the first step to overcoming them.

YOUR MENOPAUSE MAKEOVER CONTACTS

Keep a list of all Menopause Makeover contacts. Include everyone from your doctor (gynecologist, eye doctor, dentist, dermatologist) to the lab, pharmacy, health food store, practitioner, hairstylist, exercise location, trainer and your spiritual or support group.

Name	Phone Number	E-mail	Address

MENOPAUSE MAKEOVER MEDICAL FORMS

CURRENT EMOTIONAL AND PHYSICAL CONCERNS

List your current emotional and physical concerns, such as vision changes, skin issues, high blood pressure, weight gain, migraines, hair loss, mood swings, depression, fatigue, panic attacks, difficulty with sex and low libido.

1.

2.

3.

4.

5.

6.

7.

8.

9.

10.

YOUR PERSONAL MEDICAL HISTORY

Document YOUR medical history.

EXAMPLE: Pregnancy complications, allergies, migraines, high blood pressure, endometriosis, fibroids, diabetes, broken bones, past surgeries, injuries, fatigue, seizures, asthma, infertility, incontinence, losing height, hair loss, dizziness, hospitalization, mental health problems, cancer, arthritis, history of smoking.

YOUR FAMILY MEDICAL HISTORY

Genetics can affect treatment choices and offer you the opportunity to prevent future problems. Discuss your family medical history with your doctor. What diseases run in your family? Check off all those that apply.

- Heart disease
- High blood pressure
- Glaucoma
- Blood clots
- Stroke
- Elevated cholesterol
- Breast cancer
- Uterine cancer
- Ovarian cancer
- Fibroids
- Kidney problems
- Depression
- Diabetes
- Allergies
- Alzheimer's
- Arthritis

- Challenging menopause
- Chronic fatigue
- Osteoporosis
- Migraines
- Endocrine issues
- Memory loss
- Hair loss
- Obesity
- Endometriosis
- Thyroid problems
- Alcoholism/Drug Abuse
- Incontinence
- Bladder problems
- Hysterectomy
- Gallbladder disease

Other cancers:
....

Autoimmune disease (please specify):
....

List any other genetic diseases that run in your family:

....

CURRENT MEDICATIONS

List Medications (both Prescription and Over-the-counter), Vitamins, Minerals and Herbs You Currently Take.

1.

2.

3.

4.

5.

6.

7.

8.

9.

10.

11.

12.

13.

14.

15.

MEDICAL SCREENING

Are You Current With Medical Tests?

30'S	
MONTHLY	Breast self-exam
YEARLY	Annual physical; pelvic exam; check blood pressure; update necessary vaccinations; dental checkup.
EVERY 2 TO 3 YEARS	Pap smear, unless there has been a history of abnormal results or increased risk. If so, get a Pap smear every year.
EVERY 5 YEARS	Cholesterol levels and/or diabetes test, depending on your family history and risk factors.
AT THE AGE OF 35	Have your first mammogram if breast cancer runs in your family. Also consider having a thyroid test to establish a baseline.
40'S	
MONTHLY	Breast self-exam; skin self-exam — check for irregular moles.
SEMI-ANNUALLY	Dental checkup.

YEARLY	Annual physical; pelvic exam; rectal exam; update necessary vaccinations; mammogram; blood pressure screening; cholesterol profile; a thyroid test, if needed. Diabetes screening if indicated by personal or family history.
EVERY 2 TO 3 YEARS	Pap smear, unless there has been a history of abnormal results. If so, get a Pap smear every year; eye exam.

50's

MONTHLY	Breast self-exam; skin self-exam—check for irregular moles.
SEMI-ANNUALLY	Dental checkup.
YEARLY	Annual physical; pelvic exam; rectal exam; check blood pressure; update necessary vaccinations; mammogram; cholesterol levels. Bone density test if indicated by risk factors.
EVERY 2 TO 3 YEARS	Pap smear, unless there has been a history of abnormal results. If so, get a Pap smear every year.

EVERY 5 YEARS	Colon screening (colonoscopy) when you turn 50. If your colon screening is normal, have one every 5 to 10 years, depending on your personal risk factors.

60's

MONTHLY	Breast self-exam; skin self-exam —check for irregular moles.
SEMI-ANNUALLY	Dental checkup.
YEARLY	Annual physical; pelvic exam; check blood pressure; update necessary vaccinations; rectal exam; mammogram. Check cholesterol levels.
EVERY 1 TO 2 YEARS	Eye exam and glaucoma test.
EVERY 2 TO 3 YEARS	Pap smear, unless there has been a history of abnormal results. If so, get a Pap smear every year.
ONCE YOU ARE 65	Bone density test. Get a shingles vaccine (only needed once), and a pneumonia vaccine every 10 years starting at 65. Get a flu shot every year.

70's

MONTHLY	Breast self-exam; skin self-exam –check for irregular moles.
SEMI-ANNUALLY	Dental checkup.
YEARLY	Annual physical; pelvic exam; check blood pressure and cholesterol levels.
EVERY 1 TO 2 YEARS	Eye exam and glaucoma test; colonoscopy every 5 to 10 years; mammogram.
EVERY 1 TO 3 YEARS	After age 70, you do not need a Pap smear unless indicated, but a pelvic and rectal exam are recommended.

Note: Mammogram recommendations are based on the American Cancer Society guidelines.

MENOPAUSE MAKEOVER FOOD PLAN

A food plan is a great way to stick to your Makeover!
Use the sample plan to create your own customized
food plan on page 354.

SAMPLE FOOD PLAN

BASED ON **1,200** CALORIES PER DAY

MON	TUES	WED	THUR
BREAKFAST			
½ cup strawberries ½ cup low-fat cottage cheese coffee	½ cup oatmeal ½ scoop protein powder ½ cup blueberries ½ cup soymilk coffee	protein shake	1 egg hardboiled 3 oz lean ham coffee
MORNING SNACK			
100-calorie protein bar	100-calorie protein shake	½ cup fruit ½ cup cottage cheese	100-calorie protein bar

FRI	SAT	SUN
BREAKFAST		
$\frac{1}{2}$ cup fruit $\frac{1}{2}$ cup cottage cheese coffee	low-fat yogurt coffee	baked frittata (see recipe)
MORNING SNACK		
100-calorie protein shake	100-calorie protein bar	$\frac{1}{2}$ cup fruit $\frac{1}{2}$ cup cottage cheese

	MON	TUES	WED	THUR
LUNCH				
	1 cup veggie 6 oz grilled chicken breast (meat only, grilled or broiled)	4 oz tuna $\frac{1}{2}$ whole wheat pita pocket light mayo $\frac{1}{2}$ cup fruit	1 cup lean turkey chili 1 medium apple	crabmeat pita $\frac{1}{2}$ whole wheat pita pocket 4 oz crabmeat, 1 tsp light mayo
AFTERNOON SNACK				
	low-fat string cheese	1 oz cashews 1 small apple	mocha shake (see recipe)	1 oz macadamia nuts
DINNER				
	6 oz pork chop 1 cup broccoli $\frac{1}{2}$ cup couscous	6 oz grilled salmon 1 cup veggie baby lettuce & 1 tbsp low-fat dressing	6 oz chicken grilled 1 cup veggie $\frac{1}{2}$ cup brown rice	6 oz halibut 1 cup asparagus 1 cup wild rice
EVENING SNACK				
	low-fat yogurt	3.5 oz red wine low-fat string cheese	2 oz turkey lunch meat small pear	protein shake

FRI	SAT	SUN
		LUNCH
chicken salad 6 oz grilled chicken & lettuce with veggies	1 veggie burger 1 slice of whole wheat bread	chicken curry salad (see recipe) sparkling water
		AFTERNOON SNACK
4 oz tuna, light mayo, 2 melba toasts	low-fat string cheese ½ cup fruit	2 hardboiled eggs stuffed with hummus sprinkle paprika for spice
		DINNER
6 oz pork tenderloin salad with low-fat dressing	chicken & veggie fondue (see recipe) lettuce & 1 tbsp low-fat dressing 6 oz white wine	stir-fry chicken & veggies small salad
		EVENING SNACK
fruit low-fat string cheese	fruit & low-fat yogurt	100-calorie protein bar

FOOD PLAN

BASED ON _____ CALORIES PER DAY

	MON	TUES	WED	THUR
BREAKFAST				
MORNING SNACK				
LUNCH				
AFTERNOON SNACK				
DINNER				
EVENING SNACK				

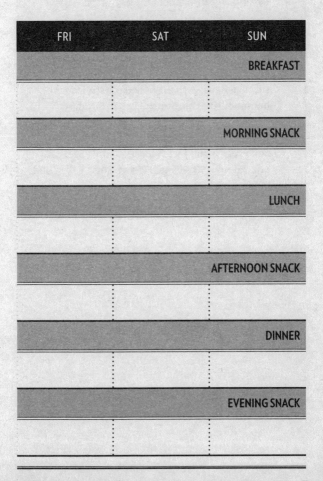

FRI	SAT	SUN	
			BREAKFAST
			MORNING SNACK
			LUNCH
			AFTERNOON SNACK
			DINNER
			EVENING SNACK

MAKEOVER TIPS

- Don't let four hours pass without eating.

- Drink water throughout the day.

- Eat protein with each meal and most snacks.

- If you "crash" (blood sugar drops from waiting too long to eat), grab one of these snacks: fruits, low-fat string cheese, low-fat cottage cheese, sliced deli turkey, hard-boiled egg stuffed with hummus, 100-calorie protein bar, 5 Nabisco™ Nilla Wafers, ½ cup of sorbet with ½ cup berries, 25 pistachios, 1 Yoplait™ light smoothie, 1 hard-boiled egg with 1 melba toast, ½ mini bagel with 1 oz. salmon, 50 edamame (soybeans), celery and hummus dip.

MENOPAUSE MAKEOVER SHOPPING LIST

Once you've determined your food plan, create a shopping list to stock your fridge with everything you need to meet your goals. Check off the foods you need in each category.

PROTEIN

- [ ] Fish & shellfish
- [ ] White-meat poultry
- [ ] Low-fat milk
- [ ] Low-fat yogurt
- [ ] Low-fat cottage cheese
- [ ] Low-fat cheese
- [ ] Eggs
- [ ] Egg whites
- [ ] Beans
- [ ] Pork tenderloin
- [ ] Soy
- [ ] Lean beef
- [ ] Protein shake
- [ ] Protein bar

Other [ ]

FATS

- [ ] Nuts (almonds, walnuts, cashews)
- [ ] Fish (salmon, halibut, flounder, crab, tuna, trout)
- [ ] Peanuts
- [ ] Avocado
- [ ] Olives
- [ ] Olive oil
- [ ] Safflower oil
- [ ] Flaxseed oil

Other [ ]

CARBOHYDRATES

☐	Legumes (kidney beans, lentils, pinto beans, chickpeas)	☐	Plain yogurt
☐	Fruit (apples, plums, oranges, raisins)	☐	Skim milk
		☐	Soy beverage
☐	Veggies (broccoli, yams, sweet potato)	☐	Brown rice
		☐	Basmati rice
☐	Fruit juices without added sugar	☐	Couscous
		☐	Rice cakes
☐	Bran cereal	☐	Whole-grain breads
☐	Oatmeal	☐	Whole-grain pasta
☐	Oat bran	☐	Rye bread
☐	All-bran		
☐	Shredded wheat cereal		

Other ☐

HIGH-FIBER FOODS

☐	Celery	☐	Oat Bran
☐	Apples	☐	Nuts
☐	Strawberries	☐	Rice Bran
☐	Blueberries	☐	Peas
☐	Pears	☐	Carrots
☐	Lentils	☐	Cucumbers
☐	Oatmeal	☐	Tomatoes

- [ ] Zucchini
- [ ] Whole-wheat breads
- [ ] Brown rice
- [ ] Barley
- [ ] Whole-wheat couscous

- [ ] Rye
- [ ] Cabbage
- [ ] Brussels sprouts
- [ ] Cauliflower
- [ ] Beets

Other [ ]

BEVERAGES

- [ ] Water
- [ ] Fruit juices without added sugar

- [ ] Coffee
- [ ] Red wine

Other [ ]

SUPPLEMENTS

- [ ] Calcium/vitamin D
- [ ] Multivitamin

- [ ] Omega-3

Other [ ]

LOW-CALORIE SNACKS

- [ ] 100-calorie cookies

- [ ] 100-calorie Popsicle®

Other [ ]

PROTEIN-RICH SNACKS

- [ ] Protein shakes

- [ ] Protein bars

Other [ ]

MENOPAUSE MAKEOVER DAILY MEAL PLAN

GOAL: 40% Protein; 35% Carbs; 25% Fats per serving

BREAKFAST

Time: _____ (Eat within one hour of waking.) List foods below

....

....

....

LUNCH

Time: _____ List foods below

....

....

....

AFTERNOON SNACK

Time: _____ List foods below

....

....

....

DINNER

Time: _____ List foods below

....

....

....

		TOTALS		
CALORIE	PROTEIN	CARBS	FAT	FIBER

GOAL: 40% Protein; 35% Carbs; 25% Fats per serving

EVENING SNACK

Time: _____ (Eat 2 hours before bedtime.) List foods below

....

....

....

TOTALS FOR THE DAY

FOOD SERVINGS

FOOD	SERVINGS PER DAY	PORTION SIZE
Protein	5-6	Size of your palm
Carbs	3-5	1 slice or 1.2 cup
Fruits	2-5	med., $^1/_2$ cup chopped, $^1/_2$ cup juice
Vegetables	3-5	1 cup raw or $^1/_2$ cup cooked
Fats	5-6	Size of your thumb
Dairy	2, nonfat	$^1/_2$ cup
Protein snacks	1-2 per day	Power bar or shake, protein powder
Water	6-8	8 fluid ounces
Coffee	Less than 2	1 cup
Alcohol	Less than 6 ounces	

TOTALS

CALORIE	PROTEIN	CARBS	FAT	FIBER

SUPPLEMENTS CHECKLIST

CALCIUM (600 mg two times a day)	VITAMIN D (400 IU two times a day)	MULTIVITAMIN
☐ ____	☐ ____	☐ ____
☐ ____	☐ ____	☐ ____

DAILY CALORIES CONSUMED

FOOD CALORIES	−	EXERCISE CALORIES	−	ACTIVITY CALORIES	=	DAILY CALORIES CONSUMED
____		____		____		____

YOUR **12**-WEEK PLAN

WEEK	1	2	3	4	5	6	7	8	9	10	11	12

Date _____   Day of Week _____

Starting Weight _____   Current Weight _____   Goal Weight _____

HORMONES (record daily)

ESTROGEN	AM	PM	PROGESTERONE	AM	PM

Monthly cycle ☐ YES ☐ NO

_____

Current medications

_____

What menopause symptoms are you experiencing?

_____

How do you feel emotionally today?

_____

EXERCISE

CARDIO | Goal > 20-30 minutes a day, 5-6 days a week.	STRENGTH BUILDING | Goal > 2-3 times per week or daily.
Weekly goal:	What type of exercise:
What type of exercise:	Intensity: ☐ low ☐ medium ☐ high
Intensity: ☐ low ☐ medium ☐ high	For how long:
For how long:	Heart-rate average:
	Did I succeed? ☐ yes ☐ no
Heart-rate average:	Calories burned:
Did I succeed? ☐ yes ☐ no	Time of day:
Calories burned:	Other Activity:
Time of day:	Calories burned:

YOUR WEEKLY PROGRESS

Date .... Day of Week ....

Starting Weight .... Current Weight .... Goal Weight ....

Weight difference from last week:

....
....

If your weight is less than last week, to what do you attribute this success? Cutting portions? Counting calories? Cutting out junk food? More exercise? Symptom treatment?

....
....
....

If your weight is more than last week, why?

What was the most difficult part of your makeover last week?

How are your menopausal symptoms?   ☐ the same ☐ better ☐ worse
How are you addressing your symptoms?

What do you enjoy most about your exercise routine?

What do you dislike about your exercise routine?

What can you do to make your exercise program more successful or enjoyable?

Have you noticed a pattern in your eating habits that you need to change?
☐ yes ☐ no
What do you need to change in your meal planning to meet your goals?

Where do you excel with your meal planning?

Where do you fall short in your meal planning?

What are your exercise and eating goals for the upcoming week?

Overall, how would you rate your emotional health this past week?

What beauty goals did you accomplish this week?

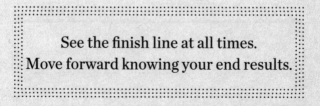

See the finish line at all times.
Move forward knowing your end results.

YOUR GRATITUDE LIST

List everything for which you are grateful. Continue
to add throughout your Menopause Makeover.

This is your chance to live your dreams.

THE MENOPAUSE MAKEOVER REWARD

Tape a photograph of your
Menopause Makeover reward here.

JOURNAL PAGES

NOTES

chapter 14

Menopause Makeover
Recipes and Menus

One of the biggest adjustments you need to make to be successful with your Menopause Makeover is creating new eating habits. What foods you eat can make the difference between a smooth menopause transition and a bumpy road. The Menopause Makeover Food Pyramid allows you the flexibility to eat delicious foods while improving your health and helping you lose weight. I have included a few of my favorite recipes to demonstrate how eating according to the food pyramid can still be incredibly satisfying and delicious. There is also room to add your own favorite makeover recipes that honor the food pyramid. Have fun with food! Be creative, and bon appetite.

FAVORITE MAKEOVER BREAKFASTS

BAKED BREAKFAST FRITTATA

The level of protein and fiber will keep you feeling full for hours. This meal honors the Menopause Makeover Food Pyramid—it is perfectly balanced, low in calories and a great way to start the day.

Servings = 6–8   Prep time = 30 minutes

1 tablespoon olive oil

$1\frac{1}{2}$ cups potatoes cut in $\frac{1}{2}$-inch cubes

$1\frac{1}{2}$ cups chopped cooked lean ham (8 oz.)

$\frac{3}{4}$-cup (3 oz.) low-fat shredded cheddar cheese

8 eggs slightly beaten (or two 8-oz. cartons of egg product)

$\frac{1}{3}$ cup low-fat milk

Chili peppers

2 teaspoons fresh oregano

$\frac{1}{4}$ teaspoon salt

4-oz. can diced green onions

2 teaspoons of psyllium husks (you can buy this powdered fiber—it has no taste—at a health food store or a grocery store like Whole Foods™)

$\frac{1}{2}$ of a 7-oz. jar of roasted red sweet peppers cut into thin strips

$1\frac{1}{2}$ cups salsa

$\frac{1}{4}$ cup fresh cilantro

3 sprigs of parsley

DIRECTIONS

- Preheat oven to 350ºF.
- In a 10-inch, oven-safe skillet, cook the potatoes in hot olive oil, uncovered over medium heat for 5 minutes. Stir occasionally. Then cover and cook for another 5 minutes until tender.
- Remove from heat and mix in the ham and $\frac{1}{2}$ cup of cheddar cheese.
- In a mixing bowl, stir together the eggs, milk, chili peppers, oregano, salt, onions and psyllium husks. Then pour into the skillet and mix together. Lay the pepper strips on top of the frittata.
- Bake uncovered for 25–30 minutes.
- Sprinkle the top with $\frac{1}{4}$ cup of cheddar cheese. In a separate pan, stir salsa and cilantro together and heat.
- Cut the frittata into wedges, place the parsley as decoration next to the wedge and serve with the salsa mixture. Serve on a smaller dish with a lovely wineglass filled with chilled water and a twist of lemon.

Calories: 196 / Carbs: 11 g / Protein: 17 g / Fiber: 2 g / Fat: 8 g

COFFEE MOCHA PROTEIN SHAKE

1 cup low-fat soy milk or fat-free milk

2 scoops of whey chocolate protein powder

2 teaspoons instant coffee, or a shot of espresso

1 teaspoon of vanilla extract

1 cup ice cubes

DIRECTIONS

- In a blender, combine all ingredients and blend until smooth. Enjoy!

Using Low-Fat Soy Milk —Calories: 243 / Carbs: 15.9 g
Protein: 29.2 g / Fiber: 4.2 g / Fat: 6.6 g
Using Fat-Free Milk —Calories: 206 / Carbs: 16.7 g / Protein: 28.3 g
Fiber: 1 g / Fat: 1.7 g

MAKEOVER TIPS

You can premake this shake and refrigerate, then pour it into an insulated thermos, so it will be ready to enjoy midafternoon.

FAVORITE MAKEOVER LUNCHES

Once you add the lettuce, pita or wrap, this meal honors the Menopause Makeover Food Pyramid food ratios of 35% protein, 40% carbohydrates and 25% fats. This yummy recipe helps you fight the menopause midsection and love handles!

By using curry, this scrumptious recipe contains enhanced health benefits. Curry is a blend of various spices, with the most common mixture being turmeric, ground cumin, cardamom and coriander. Curry boasts anti-inflammatory properties and can help promote neurological health.

With the addition of other healthy ingredients, such as onions, apples and chicken (an excellent lean meat choice), this salad is healthy yet delicious.

I like to serve this salad with sliced, chilled pears or apples on the side, and sparkling water with a sprig of mint…yummy!

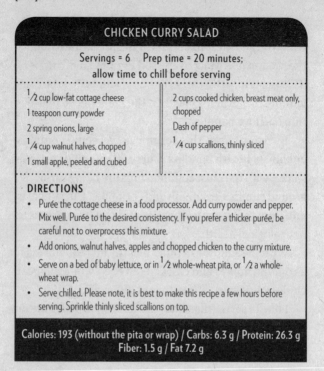

CHICKEN CURRY SALAD

Servings = 6   Prep time = 20 minutes;
allow time to chill before serving

$^1/_2$ cup low-fat cottage cheese

1 teaspoon curry powder

2 spring onions, large

$^1/_4$ cup walnut halves, chopped

1 small apple, peeled and cubed

2 cups cooked chicken, breast meat only, chopped

Dash of pepper

$^1/_4$ cup scallions, thinly sliced

DIRECTIONS

- Purée the cottage cheese in a food processor. Add curry powder and pepper. Mix well. Purée to the desired consistency. If you prefer a thicker purée, be careful not to overprocess this mixture.

- Add onions, walnut halves, apples and chopped chicken to the curry mixture.

- Serve on a bed of baby lettuce, or in $^1/_2$ whole-wheat pita, or $^1/_2$ a whole-wheat wrap.

- Serve chilled. Please note, it is best to make this recipe a few hours before serving. Sprinkle thinly sliced scallions on top.

Calories: 193 (without the pita or wrap) / Carbs: 6.3 g / Protein: 26.3 g
Fiber: 1.5 g / Fat 7.2 g

This is my all-time favorite chili recipe. The good news is that chili is not only comfort food, but it can be healthy, too! Chili contains lots of protein. (This recipe is made with turkey, so it is a leaner alternative to ground beef.) And chili can help you lose weight. "Capsaicin," a colorless compound found in the chilies used to season this dish, can increase your metabolic rate by increasing your body heat production. This recipe is also high in iron, thanks to the turkey and beans, and has vitamin C, thanks to the tomatoes, peppers and chilies. Plus, it's a great source of fiber that helps keep you full for a long time after eating. Enjoy the healthy benefits of chili!

TURKEY CHILI

Servings = 8–10   Prep time = 30 minutes

2 medium onions, chopped (1 cup)
1 tablespoon vegetable oil
2 tablespoons chopped fresh garlic
1 medium red bell pepper, chopped (1 cup)
1 medium green bell pepper, chopped (1 cup)
2 pounds ground turkey
2 tablespoons ground cumin
1 tablespoon dried oregano leaves
1 tablespoon chili powder
1 can (4 oz.) chopped green chilies, drained
2 jalapeño chilies, seeded and chopped

28-oz. can of whole Roma (plum) tomatoes
Salt and pepper to taste
3 cups water for thick meaty chili, or 4 cups for "soupier" chili
2 cans (15 oz.) black beans, drained
1 can (15–16 oz.) kidney beans, drained
Sweet onions, sliced
Low-fat sour cream

DIRECTIONS

- Cook the onions in vegetable oil in a large saucepan over medium heat for about 10 minutes or until the onions are tender.
- Add garlic and the green and red bell peppers, cook 2–3 minutes.
- Add turkey and cook 3–4 minutes or until the turkey is no longer pink.
- Add cumin, oregano leaves, chili powder, green chilies, jalapeño chilies, tomatoes, salt, pepper and water. Reduce heat to low.
- Cover and simmer about 30 minutes.
- Add beans; simmer 15–20 minutes longer. Simmer for a total of 2 hours for a rich flavor.
- To serve, add sliced sweet onions to the top and a dab of low-fat sour cream.

If you want to make this recipe spicy, add one whole red habañero or one whole serrano chili (deveined, deseeded and chopped). Or if you like a Tex-Mex flavor, add an envelope of taco seasoning as you simmer this recipe.

Calories: 175 / Carbs: 13 g / Protein: 15 g / Fiber: 5 g / Fat: 6 g

FAVORITE MAKEOVER DINNERS

ROMANTIC DINNER FOR TWO

This is a fun romantic meal—it not only helps with Step 2 of your makeover, but it will help rekindle the romance for Step 6, too!

The menu

- Tempting beginning: Chilled grapes and fruit.
- Main course: Chicken and veggie fondue with dipping sauces.
- Sinful endings: Strawberries dipped in dark chocolate.
- Wine: Red (Zinfandel).

After you have enjoyed cooking your fondue dinner, bring out the dark chocolate or chocolate-dipped strawberries for a sinful ending. Healthy dark chocolate has a cocoa content of 60–70 percent or higher. Eating 2 ounces (50 grams) a day of plain chocolate with a minimum content of 60 percent chocolate solids, can be beneficial to your health—providing protection against heart disease, high blood pressure and many other health hazards, as well as providing vitamins, and essential trace elements and nutrients, such as iron, calcium and potassium. A 1½-ounce square of chocolate may have as many cancer-fighting antioxidants as a 5-ounce glass of red wine. And chocolate stimulates the secretion of endorphins, producing a pleasurable sensation. So don't feel guilty! Enjoy some dark chocolate!

Don't forget to play your favorite music, light plenty of candles and mist yourself with sensual perfume.

CHICKEN AND VEGGIE FONDUE WITH DIPPING SAUCES

This dinner is low in fat and high in protein.
Servings = 2 Prep time = 15 minutes

1 pound skinless and boneless chicken breasts

2 cups cauliflower

2 cups broccoli

dipping sauces

DIRECTIONS

- Cut the chicken breasts and vegetables into bite-size portions.
- Place the chicken in a serving dish separate from the vegetables. Refrigerate until ready to serve.
- Place your favorite dipping sauces in separate serving dishes.

SUGGESTED DIPPING SAUCES

Peppercorn, honey-mustard, peanut satay, sesame garlic, BBQ and/or teriyaki sauce. Purchase these sauces premade and keep your special evening simple.

Remember to dip, not scoop.

FONDUE PREPARATION

- Half fill the fondue pot with vegetable oil.
- Then pour the measured oil into a saucepan on the stovetop and heat the oil to 375°F. You will know the oil is ready when you drop a piece of bread in and it browns in 30 seconds.
- Pour the oil back into the fondue pot and light the burner.
- Place the chicken, vegetables and dipping sauces around the fondue pot with a grilling fork.
- Start cooking your dinner. Each piece of chicken should cook in the fondue pot 1–2 minutes.

Chicken and Veggies: Calories: 299 / Carbs: 9.8 g
Protein: 26.7 g / Fiber: 5.1 g / Fat 3.3 g
Dipping Sauces: Peppercorn sauce (4oz. serving):
Calories: 123 / Carbs: 2.0 g / Protein: 19.3 g / Fiber: 0 g / Fat 4.3 g
BBQ sauce (1 cup serving): Calories: 187.5
Carbs: 32 g / Protein: 4.5 g / Fiber: 3.0 g / Fat 4.5 g

STRAWBERRIES DIPPED IN DARK CHOCOLATE

Servings = 4   Prep time = 15 minutes

4 oz. semisweet chocolate
1 small carton of medium-sized whole strawberries

DIRECTIONS

- Microwave chocolate in a glass bowl, stopping after 30 seconds, then every 10 seconds until almost melted.
- Stir until smooth and glossy.
- Wash strawberries and pat them dry (any moisture from the fruit will spoil the texture of the melted chocolate).
- Dip each strawberry into the melted chocolate, covering the lower half of the strawberry.
- Place on a baking sheet lined with wax paper.
- Refrigerate for at least 1 hour.

Per chocolate strawberry—Calories: 48 / Carbs: 6.8 g
Protein: 0.5 g / Fiber: 1.1 g / Fat: 18 g

Tips for Selecting Your Wine

- The wine should not be sweeter than the chocolate you are serving.
- When pairing wines with chocolate, the stronger the chocolate, the more full-bodied the wine should be. For example, a bittersweet chocolate tends to pair well with an intense Zinfandel.

ROASTED TURKEY

This recipe is perfect for entertaining, or makes a great dinner for two with healthy leftovers.   Servings = 10–12

12–14 pound whole turkey, giblets removed

A couple sprigs each of fresh thyme, oregano, sage and parsley

3 tablespoons olive oil

2 tablespoons dry white wine

2 tablespoons paprika

Fresh ground pepper to taste

3 small oranges, unpeeled and cut into wedges

2 onions, cut into wedges

1 cup of low-fat, low-sodium chicken broth

DIRECTIONS

- Preheat the oven to 325°F.
- Lift up the skin covering the turkey breast.
- Slip the thyme, oregano, sage and parsley underneath the skin.
- Combine the oil, wine, paprika and pepper. Rub this mixture over the surface of the turkey.
- Place the oranges and onions inside the turkey.
- Place the turkey, breast-side down, in a roasting pan. Pour chicken broth into the bottom of the pan. Cover loosely with aluminum foil.
- Roast for 20–25 minutes per pound, basting periodically.
- Halfway through cooking, place breast-side up.
- During the last 45 minutes of roasting, remove the foil cover.
- Continue to roast until the leg moves easily and the juices run clear. (Minimal internal temperature should be 165°F, measured with a food thermometer.)
- Let stand for 20 minutes to let juices settle for easier carving.

Calories: 386 / Carbs: 4.5 g / Protein: 29.0 g / Fiber: 0.9 g / Fat: 11.5 g

ENTERTAINING IDEAS

For an elegant and easy-on-your-waistline dinner that serves 10 to 12, try:

Roasted turkey	Endive, watercress and pear salad	Acorn squash
Crudités with low-fat hummus dip	Wild rice	Baked apples

FAVORITE MAKEOVER SIDES AND SNACKS

WILD RICE

Servings = 10-12

1 cup wild rice
2 cups water

Salt and pepper to taste

DIRECTIONS

- In a pan, combine the rice and water.
- Boil, reduce heat and simmer until the rice is tender, usually 40–45 minutes.
- Drain, add salt and pepper.

Calories: 83 / Carbs: 34 g / Protein: 7 g / Fiber: 3 g / Fat: 0.2 g

LOW-FAT HUMMUS DIP

Servings = 10-12

2 cans (15 oz.) garbanzo beans,
drained; save the juice
6 teaspoons lemon juice
4 tablespoons sesame tahini

6 cloves garlic peeled
1 teaspoon salt
1/2 teaspoon pepper

DIRECTIONS

- Combine all ingredients in a blender or food processor.
- Process until smooth, and add the reserved garbanzo juice for a nice creamy texture.
- Serve with vegetables. Bell peppers, celery, cucumbers and carrots make a lovely and tasty presentation.
- This recipe makes it possible to prepare two bowls of low-fat hummus, so you can have a presentation in the living room and one in the kitchen, while your guests keep you company during the turkey preparation.

Calories: 114 / Carbs: 16.5 g / Protein: 1.4 g / Fiber: 2.8 g / Fat: 2.6 g

ACORN SQUASH

Servings = 10–12

| 5 acorn squashes, cut in half (scoop out seeds) | 1/2 cup water |

DIRECTIONS

- Preheat oven to 350°F.
- Put acorn squash halves, cut-side down, in a baking pan.
- Add water and bake under tender (usually 30–50 minutes).

Calories: 115 / Carbs: 30 g / Protein: 2 g / Fiber: 9 g / Fat: 0 g

ENDIVE, WATERCRESS AND PEAR SALAD

Servings = 10–12

Watercress, 3 large bunches, stems removed	Salt and ground pepper, to taste
Belgian endive, 3 heads, cored and separated into leaves	White balsamic vinegar (or pear vinegar), 3 tablespoons
5 tablespoons extra-virgin olive oil	3 ripe pears, halved and cored, then cut in half again lengthwise

DIRECTIONS

- In a large bowl, toss watercress and Belgian endive.
- Add extra-virgin olive oil and toss again.
- Sprinkle salt and freshly ground pepper, toss.
- Pour white balsamic vinegar, or pear vinegar, and then toss.
- Garnish your salad with the pear wedges. Serve immediately.

Calories: 100 / Carbs: 11.2 g / Protein: 2 g / Fiber: 5 g / Fat: 6.3 g

FAVORITE MAKEOVER DESSERTS

BAKED APPLES

My husband taught me this delicious recipe. It's an old family favorite!   Servings = 10-12

12 tart Jonathon apples

1 $\frac{1}{2}$ cups brown sugar

12 tablespoons light margarine (Smart Balance Light™)

6 teaspoons ground cinnamon

DIRECTIONS

- Preheat oven to 350°F.
- Core the apples but leave the bottom intact, so it looks like a "well" in the apple.
- Prick the apple skins with a fork so the apple can "breathe" while baking.
- Fill the hole with 2 tablespoons of brown sugar and 1 tablespoon of margarine.
- Then place the apples in a baking dish with a thin layer of water on the bottom, and sprinkle each apple with cinnamon.
- Bake for 20 minutes (10 minutes covered with foil and 10 minutes uncovered) until the apples are tender and begin to caramelize.

You can also add chopped walnuts or pecans to the "stuffing."

And you may want to top this yummy recipe with a low-fat frozen vanilla yogurt.

Calories: 252 / Carbs: 51 g / Protein: 0.1 g / Fiber: 5.8 g / Fat: 8.1 g

YOUR FAVORITE MAKEOVER RECIPES

Insert your favorite recipes for easy reference.

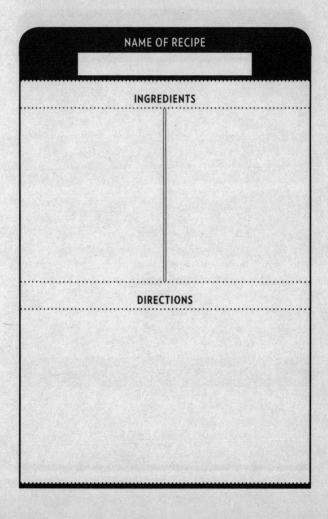

NAME OF RECIPE

INGREDIENTS

DIRECTIONS

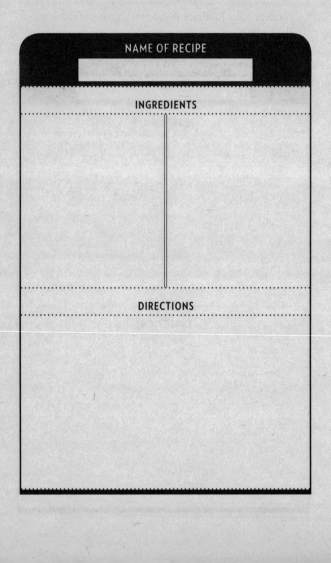

NAME OF RECIPE

INGREDIENTS

DIRECTIONS

chapter 15

You've Just Begun

You have just completed the Menopause Makeover. Congratulations! You have started creating the new you. Do you like what you see? Do you feel good? Is there room for improvement? Was your Makeover so incredible that you want to relax and enjoy your successes? Is it time for another party?

This is the Menopause Makeover debriefing chapter! After you complete your Makeover, you have a number of possibilities.

- Repeat the 12-Week Plan with revised goals.
- Repeat the 12-Week Plan with the same goals, so you have extra time to achieve your results.
- Start a support group with other menopausal gals and share your secrets.
- Start a support group and do the Menopause Makeover as a team.
- Share your success story online at www.menopausemakeover.com.

AFTER YOUR MAKEOVER

HOW DO YOU FEEL AFTER YOUR MENOPAUSE MAKEOVER?

Did you achieve most of your goals?   ☐ yes   ☐ no
....

What specific results did you accomplish?

```
..................................................................................
:                                                                                :
:                                                                                :
:                                                                                :
:                                                                                :
..................................................................................
```

Overall, in what area(s) did you excel? Check all that apply:
☐ hormones   ☐ nutrition   ☐ exercise   ☐ beauty
☐ emotions   ☐ relationships   ☐ spirituality   ☐ happiness

What area needs improvement?
```
..................................................................................
:                                                                                :
:                                                                                :
:                                                                                :
..................................................................................
```

Do you need to reset your goals?   ☐ yes   ☐ no
....

Were you too ambitious?   ☐ yes   ☐ no
....

Not ambitious enough?   ☐ yes   ☐ no
....

Did you get support from friends and loved ones? ☐ yes ☐ no

Do you feel prettier after your makeover? ☐ yes ☐ no

Do you feel happier after your makeover? ☐ yes ☐ no

Do you feel better about your body? ☐ yes ☐ no

Do you have fewer menopausal symptoms? ☐ yes ☐ no

Are you working closely with your health-care practitioner to
achieve menopausal health? ☐ yes ☐ no

Did you create an exercise program that you enjoy and that
fits into your lifestyle? ☐ yes ☐ no

Did you honor your weekly food plans? ☐ yes ☐ no

What are you most thankful about after completing your makeover?

What relationships improved?

Are your emotions more stable?   ☐ N/A ☐ yes ☐ no

....

What symptoms still need attention?

What symptoms disappeared?

What new beauty goal are you enjoying most?

Have you grown as a person over the past 12 weeks?   ☐ yes ☐ no

....

Are you pursuing your goals daily?   ☐ yes ☐ no

....

What did you enjoy most during the 12-Week Plan?

When you repeat the Menopause Makeover, what one thing would you change?

Did you meet your goals for:

Health	☐ yes ☐ no	Emotions	☐ yes ☐ no
Hormones	☐ yes ☐ no	Relationships	☐ yes ☐ no
Nutrition	☐ yes ☐ no	Spirituality	☐ yes ☐ no
Exercise	☐ yes ☐ no	Happiness	☐ yes ☐ no
Beauty	☐ yes ☐ no		

Rate each area of your Menopause Makeover — 10, you excelled; 1, no results:

	EXCELLED 10	9	8	7	6	5	4	3	2	1	NO RESULTS
Health	○	○	○	○	○	○	○	○	○	○	Health
Hormones	○	○	○	○	○	○	○	○	○	○	Hormones
Nutrition	○	○	○	○	○	○	○	○	○	○	Nutrition
Exercise	○	○	○	○	○	○	○	○	○	○	Exercise
Beauty	○	○	○	○	○	○	○	○	○	○	Beauty
Emotions	○	○	○	○	○	○	○	○	○	○	Emotions
Relationships	○	○	○	○	○	○	○	○	○	○	Relationships
Spirituality	○	○	○	○	○	○	○	○	○	○	Spirituality
Happiness	○	○	○	○	○	○	○	○	○	○	Happiness
	EXCELLED 10	9	8	7	6	5	4	3	2	1	NO RESULTS

How can you improve in each area?

Health

Hormones

Nutrition

Exercise

Beauty

Emotions

Relationships

Spirituality

Happiness

In what area is improvement impossible?

Why?

Are you willing to move forward without improvement in this area?

☐ yes   ☐ no

Do you need professional support in this area?

What habits do you need to change so you can achieve your goals?

What behavior is holding you back?

How can you change it, so you can achieve your goals?

What lessons did you learn from your Menopause Makeover?

What are you most excited about after completing your Menopause Makeover?

When will you enjoy your Menopause Makeover reward?

REPEATING THE 12-WEEK PLAN AND SETTING NEW GOALS

What results do you want to achieve for the next 12-Week Plan?

Health

Hormones

Nutrition

Exercise

Beauty

Emotions

Relationships

Spirituality

Happiness

If the goals are the same, what will you change to accomplish your goals?

If the goals are different, how will you stay motivated?

What is your greatest hope for the next 12-Week Plan?

::
.
.
.
.
.
::

What is your greatest fear?

::
.
.
.
.
::

How will you overcome this fear?

::
.
.
.
.
::

Do you need support to be successful?   ☐ yes   ☐ no

What is your action plan for the next 12 weeks?

::
.
.
.
::

What reward will you give yourself when you complete the next 12-Week Plan?

::
.
.
.
::

FUTURE GOALS

How could your life be better?

Are you willing to make changes to achieve this goal?   ☐ yes   ☐ no

Incorporate all future goals into your next Menopause Makeover. The tracking process in the 12-Week Essential Planner can be used to accomplish *all* your goals. You can personalize each 12-week session to meet your specific goals.

START YOUR OWN MENOPAUSE SUPPORT GROUP

Accountability is one of the strongest motivators for achieving goals. Millions of women are in one of the stages of menopause in the United States. Since *you* have completed the Menopause Makeover, share your expertise. Begin your very own Menopause Makeover support group. Meet once a week to discuss your goals and challenges; share recipes and exercise regimens; seek emotional support. A sisterhood of menopausal women can offer understanding, information and some much-needed humor. Brainstorming for yourself and each other can be fun. A group of women with something in common can be a powerful force. Embrace your hardships and celebrate your victories.

> Each day is a new journey
> toward your powerful potential.

Your Menopause Makeover Resources

Giving back

Doing the Menopause Makeover gave me an unexpected gift. After practicing all eight steps of the Menopause Makeover (health, nutrition, exercise, beauty, emotions, relationships, spirituality and happiness) and applying them to my life, I finally felt whole and complete. This liberating freedom left me asking, "Now what?"

Looking to remarkable women, like Oprah Winfrey, for the answer, a life lesson was revealed. It was time to *give back*. Focusing on giving allowed me to add purpose to my life!

Passionate about women's health I decided to support the following organizations, because both are making a remarkable difference in women's health.

You, too, can help these incredible organizations in their mission to advance women's health. We can forge a path with new health options for our daughters. Release your *powerful potential* and make a difference in women's health.

NORTH AMERICAN MENOPAUSE SOCIETY (NAMS), the leading nonprofit scientific organization devoted to promoting women's health and quality of life through an understanding of menopause. NAMS is recognized as the preeminent resource on all aspects of menopause to both health-care providers and the public. This organization has a useful list of NAMS-certified menopause practitioners, and the latest news about menopause and hormone therapy.

For more information: www.menopause.org/

THE SOCIETY FOR WOMEN'S HEALTH RESEARCH is the nation's only nonprofit organization whose mission is to improve the health of all women through research, education and advocacy. The society encourages the study of sex differences between women and men that affect the prevention, diagnosis and treatment of disease.

For more information: www.womenshealthresearch.org

APPENDIX A

Hormone Products for Postmenopausal Use in the United States and Canada

ORAL ET PRODUCTS FOR POSTMENOPAUSAL USE IN THE UNITED STATES AND CANADA

COMPOSITION	PRODUCT NAME	AVAILABLE DOSAGES (MG)
conjugated estrogens (formerly conjugated equine estrogens)	Premarin	0.3, 0.45,* 0.625, 0.9, 1.25
synthetic conjugated estrogens, A	Cenestin*	0.3, 0.45, 0.625, 0.9, 1.25
	Congest**	0.3, 0.625, 0.9, 1.25, 2.5
	C.E.S**	0.3, 0.625, 0.9, 1.25
	PMS-Conjugated**	0.3, 0.625, 0.9, 1.25
synthetic conjugated estrogens, B	Enjuvia*	0.3, 0.45, 0.625, 0.9, 1.25
esterified estrogens	Menest*	0.3, 0.625, 1.25, 2.5
	Neo-Estrone**	0.3, 0.625, 1.25
17β-estradiol	Estrace	0.5, 1.0, 2.0
	various generics	0.5, 1.0, 2.0
estradiol acetate	Femtrace*	0.45, 0.9, 1.8
estropipate (formerly piperazine estrone sulfate)	Ortho-Est*	0.625 (0.75 estropipate, calculated as sodium estrone sulfate 0.625), 1.25 (1.5), 2.5 (3.0)
	Ogen** various generics	0.625 (0.75), 1.25 (1.5), 2.5 (3.0), 0.625 (0.75), 1.25 (3.0)

TRANSDERMAL AND TOPICAL ET PRODUCTS FOR POSTMENOPAUSAL USE IN THE UNITED STATES AND CANADA

PRODUCT NAME	DELIVERY RATE (MG/DAY)	DOSING
17ß-ESTRADIOL – MATRIX PATCH		
Alora*	0.025, 0.05, 0.075, 0.1	twice weekly
Climara	0.025, 0.0375*, 0.05, 0.075, 0.1	once weekly
Esclim*	0.025, 0.0375, 0.05, 0.075, 0.1	twice weekly
Estradot**	0.025, 0.0375, 0.05, 0.075, 0.1	twice weekly
Menostar*	0.014	once weekly
Oesclim**	0.05, 0.1	twice weekly
Vivelle	0.05, 0.1*	twice weekly
Vivelle-Dot*	0.025, 0.0375, 0.05, 0.075, 0.1	twice weekly
various generics	0.1, 0.05	once or twice weekly
17ß-ESTRADIOL – RESERVOIR PATCH		
Estraderm	0.05, 0.1	twice weekly (patch cannot be cut)

TRANSDERMAL AND TOPICAL ET PRODUCTS FOR POSTMENOPAUSAL USE IN THE UNITED STATES AND CANADA

PRODUCT NAME	DELIVERY RATE (MG/DAY)	DOSING
17β-ESTRADIOL — TRANSDERMAL GEL		
EstroGel	0.06%*, 0.035	daily application; 1 metered pump delivers 1.25 g of gel containing 0.75 mg 17β-estradiol
Estrogel	0.06%**	daily application; 1 metered pump delivers 1.25 g of gel containing 0.75 mg 17β-estradiol
Elestrin	0.06%*, 0.0125	daily application; 1 metered pump delivers 0.87 g of gel containing 0.52 mg 17β-estradiol
17β-ESTRADIOL — TRANSDERMAL GEL		
Divigel 0.1%*	0.003, 0.009, 0.027	daily application; 3 strengths of packets provide 0.25, 0.5, or 1.0 g of gel

TRANSDERMAL AND TOPICAL ET PRODUCTS FOR POSTMENOPAUSAL USE IN THE UNITED STATES AND CANADA

PRODUCT NAME	DELIVERY RATE (MG/DAY)	DOSING
17ß-ESTRADIOL — PACKETS; TOPICAL EMULSION		
Estrasorb*	0.05 (2 packets)	daily application of 2 1 packet = 1.74 g of emulsion
17ß-ESTRADIOL — TRANSDERMAL SPRAY		
Evamist*	0.021 mg per 90 mcL spray (metered-dose pump)	initial: 1 spray/day of 1.7% solution, increasing to 2-3 sprays/day if needed

Chart copyright © 2009 The North American Menopause Society. All rights reserved. Used with permission.

*Available in the United States but not Canada.
**Available in Canada but not the United States.
Products not marked with one or two asterisks are available in both the United States and Canada.

VAGINAL ET PRODUCTS FOR POSTMENOPAUSAL USE IN THE UNITED STATES AND CANADA

COMPOSITION	PRODUCT NAME	DOSING
VAGINAL CREAMS		
17ß-estradiol	Estrace Vaginal Cream*	initial: 2–4 g/day for 1–2 wk maintenance: 1 g/day (0.1 mg active ingredient/g)
conjugated estrogens (formerly conjugated equine estrogens)	Premarin Vaginal Cream	0.5-2 g/day (0.625 mg active ingredient/g)
esterified estrogens	Neo-Estrone Vaginal Cream**	2-4 g/day (1 mg active ingredient/g)
VAGINAL RINGS		
17ß-estradiol	Estring	device containing 2 mg releases 7.5 µg/day for 90 days
estradiol acetate	Femring*	device containing 12.4 mg or 24.8 mg estradiol acetate releases 0.05 mg/day or 0.10 mg/day estradiol for 90 days (systemic levels)

VAGINAL ET PRODUCTS FOR POSTMENOPAUSAL USE IN THE UNITED STATES AND CANADA

COMPOSITION	PRODUCT NAME	DOSING
VAGINAL TABLET		
estradiol hemihydrate	Vagifem	initial: 1 tablet/day for 2 wk maintenance: 1 tablet twice/wk (tablet containing 25.8 **µ**g of estradiol hemihydrate equivalent to 25 **µ**g of estradiol)

PROGESTOGENS USED FOR EPT IN THE UNITED STATES AND CANADA

COMPOSITION	PRODUCT NAME	AVAILABLE DOSAGES
ORAL TABLET: PROGESTIN		
medroxyprogesterone acetate	Provera, various generics	2.5, 5, 10 mg
norethindrone (formerly norethisterone)	Micronor, Nor-QD,* various generics	0.35 mg
norethindrone acetate	Aygestin,* various generics	5 mg
norgestrel	Ovrette*	0.075 mg
megestrol acetate	Megace, various generics	20*, 40 mg
ORAL CAPSULE: PROGESTERONE		
progesterone (in peanut oil)	Prometrium	100, 200* mg
INTRAUTERINE SYSTEM: PROGESTIN		
levonorgestrel	Mirena	20 μg/day approx release rate (52 mg IUS has 5-yr use)

PROGESTOGENS USED FOR EPT IN THE UNITED STATES AND CANADA		
COMPOSITION	**PRODUCT NAME**	**AVAILABLE DOSAGES**
VAGINAL GEL: PROGESTERONE		
progesterone	Prochieve 4%* Crinone 4%**	45 mg/applicator

*Available in the United States but not Canada.

**Available in Canada but not the United States.

Products not marked with one or two asterisks are available in both the United States and Canada.

COMBINATION EPT PRODUCTS FOR POSTMENOPAUSAL USE IN THE UNITED STATES AND CANADA

COMPOSITION	PRODUCT NAME	AVAILABLE DOSAGES (MG/DAY)
ORAL CONTINUOUS-CYCLIC REGIMEN		
conjugated estrogens (E) + medroxyprogesterone acetate (P) (E alone for days 1–14, followed by E + P on days 15–28)	Premphase*	0.625 mg E + 5.0 mg P (2 tablets: E and E + P)
ORAL CONTINUOUS-COMBINED REGIMEN		
conjugated estrogens (E) + medroxyprogesterone acetate (P)	Prempro*	0.625 mg E + 2.5 or 5.0 mg P (1 tablet); 0.3 or 0.45 mg E + 1.5 mg P (1 tablet)
	Premplus**	0.625 mg E + 2.5 or 5.0 mg P (2 tablets: E and P)
ethinyl estradiol (E) + norethindrone acetate (P)	femhrt*	2.5 μg E + 0.5 mg P (1 tablet);
	femHRT**	5 μg E + 1mg P (1 tablet)
		5 μg E + 1 mg P (1 tablet)

COMBINATION EPT PRODUCTS FOR POSTMENOPAUSAL USE IN THE UNITED STATES AND CANADA

COMPOSITION	PRODUCT NAME	AVAILABLE DOSAGES (mg/day)
17β-estradiol (E) + norethindrone acetate (P)	Activella*	0.5 mg E + 0.1 mg P (1 tablet); 1 mg E + 0.5 mg P (1 tablet)
17β-estradiol (E) + drospirenone (P)	Angeliq*	1 mg E + 0.5 mg P (1 tablet)

ORAL INTERMITTENT-COMBINED REGIMEN

COMPOSITION	PRODUCT NAME	AVAILABLE DOSAGES (mg/day)
17β-estradiol (E) + norgestimate (P) (E alone for 3 days, followed by E+P for 3 days, repeated continuously)	Prefest*	1 mg E + 0.09 mg P (2 tablets: E and E + P)

TRANSDERMAL CONTINUOUS-COMBINED REGIMEN

COMPOSITION	PRODUCT NAME	AVAILABLE DOSAGES (mg/day)
17β-estradiol (E) + norethindrone acetate (P)	CombiPatch,*	0.05 mg E + 0.14 mg P (9 cm² patch, twice/wk)
	Estalis**	0.05 mg E + 0.25 mg P (16 cm² patch, twice/wk)
17β-estradiol (E) + levonorgestrel (P)	Climara Pro*	0.045 mg E + 0.015 mg P (22 cm² patch, once/wk)

COMBINATION EPT PRODUCTS FOR POSTMENOPAUSAL USE IN THE UNITED STATES AND CANADA

COMPOSITION	PRODUCT NAME	AVAILABLE DOSAGES (MG/DAY)
TRANSDERMAL CONTINUOUS-SEQUENTIAL REGIMEN		
17ß-estradiol (E) + norethindrone acetate (P)	Estalis Sequi**	0.05 mg E twice/wk (Vivelle 50 patch) for 2 wks, then 9 or 16 cm²
E alone for 2 wks, followed by E+P twice/wk for 2 wks, repeated continuously	Estracomb**	Estalis patch twice/wk for 2 wks
		0.05 mg E twice/wk for 2 wks, then 0.05 mg E + 0.25 mg P for 2 wks

Chart copyright © 2009 The North American Menopause Society. All rights reserved. Used with permission.

*Available in the United States but not Canada.
**Available in Canada but not the United States.

WARNING: Prometrium (micronized progesterone) is formulated in a peanut-oil suspension. If you are allergic to peanuts, you cannot take this kind of progesterone.

Supplements

BODY BENEFITS	FOOD SOURCES	DAILY DOSE	GENERAL INFO
VITAMIN A			
Treats skin disorders such as acne. Good for eye health. There are some claims that there are antioxidant benefits. Vitamin A can improve immune function.	Fish, dark colored fruits and veggies, carrots, eggs, and dairy products.	2,330 IU	Fat-soluble, stored in body. Do not take with blood thinners.
THIAMINE (B1)			
Good for the nervous system, muscle functioning, carbohydrate metabolism. Aids proper digestion.	Legumes, pork, enriched whole grains, beef, oranges, oats, milk, nuts and rice.	1.1 mg	Water-soluble; excess is excreted in the urine. Large doses may cause drowsiness.
RIBOFLAVIN (B2)			
Necessary for normal cell function.	Organ meats, milk, whole grains, eggs, green veggies, asparagus and broccoli.	1.1 mg	Water-soluble, excess is excreted in the urine. Use caution if also taking herbs and other supplements with hormonal, diuretic or antidepressant activity.

BODY BENEFITS	FOOD SOURCES	DAILY DOSE	GENERAL INFO
NIACIN (B3)			
Has been used to treat high cholesterol. May benefit age-related macular degeneration (AMD).	Fish, meat, enriched whole grains, yeast, milk, eggs and green veggies.	16-18 mg	Water-soluble, excess is excreted in the urine. B3 can precipitate hot flashes in some women. Skin flushing to the face and neck may occur. Take with a meal to avoid GI discomfort.
PANTHOTHENIC ACID (B5)			
Essential to all life, and to the metabolism of carbohydrates, proteins and fats, as well as the synthesis of hormones and cholesterol.	Brewer's yeast, organ meats, egg, fish, shellfish, poultry, veggies, legumes and milk.	5-10 mg	Water-soluble, excess is excreted in the urine. Drugs containing estrogen and progestin may increase your daily requirement.

BODY BENEFITS	FOOD SOURCES	DAILY DOSE	GENERAL INFO
PYRIDOXINE (B6)			
Required for the synthesis of the neurotransmitter serotonin. Deficiency can affect nerves, skin, mucous membranes and the blood cell system.	Meat, liver, fish, fortified cereals, beans, carrots, spinach, peas, potatoes, milk, cheese and eggs.	1.3 to 1.5 mg	Water-soluble, excess is excreted in the urine. Supplements with estrogen-like activity may interact with B6.
FOLIC ACID B9 - (ALSO KNOWN AS FOLATE)			
Often used to treat diabetes type 2, high blood pressure, insomnia and restless legs syndrome.	Liver, green leafy veggies, brewer's yeast, cereals, asparagus, OJ, bananas, melons, lemons, legumes and mushrooms.	400 mg to 1,000 mg	Water-soluble. Large doses of antacids can reduce folic acid absorption.
COBALAMIN (B12)			
Helps maintain healthy nerve cells and red blood cells.	Seafood, meat, poultry, egg yolk, dairy products, eggs and chicken.	2.4 mg	Water-soluble, excess is excreted in the urine. Excessive alcohol intake can decrease vitamin B12 absorption.

BODY BENEFITS	FOOD SOURCES	DAILY DOSE	GENERAL INFO
VITAMIN C			
Necessary to form collagen in bones, cartilage, muscle and blood vessels. There is ongoing research on the use of vitamin C in the prevention/ treatment of the common cold. There have been more than 30 clinical trials that showed no significant reduction in the risk of developing colds.	Citrus fruits, Brussels sprouts, tomatoes, broccoli, berries, bananas, alfalfa, potatoes, cantaloupe, spinach, watermelon, red and green peppers, oysters, oranges, veggies.	75 mg	Water-soluble, excess is excreted in the urine. High doses may cause diarrhea, and nausea. Oral estrogens may decrease the effect of vitamin C in the body.
VITAMIN D			
Aids in the absorption of calcium, helping to form and maintain strong bones.	5-15 minutes of sunshine can boost vitamin D production. Fish, eggs, fortified milk and cod liver oil also provide vitamin D.	400 IU taken twice a day for a total of 800 IU	Fat-soluble. Intestinal absorption of vitamin D may be impaired with the use of mineral oil.

BODY BENEFITS	FOOD SOURCES	DAILY DOSE	GENERAL INFO
VITAMIN E			
Many people claim that vitamin E may prevent cardiovascular disease and cancer. But recent studies conclude that high-doses of vitamin E (over 400 IU daily) may increase all-cause mortality and should be avoided.	Green leafy veggies, nuts, fortified cereals, vegetable oil and wheat germ.	8 mg or 12 IU	Fat-soluble, can thin blood. Do not take with blood thinners without medical supervision. Caution that vitamin E over 400 IU/day is to be avoided in people taking warfarin and related anticoagulants because it interferes with platelet function.
BORON			
May increase levels of certain estrogens.	Peanut butter, grapes, wine, peanuts, peaches.	0.96 mg	Overdose can cause nausea, vomiting, skin rash and diarrhea.
CALCIUM / CALCIUM CARBONATE			
Helps keep bones and teeth strong. Maintains muscle and nerve functioning.	Milk, yogurt, cheese, nuts, tofu, kale, broccoli and spinach.	1,200 mg; take in divided doses 2 times per day	Must take with vitamin D for absorption.

BODY BENEFITS	FOOD SOURCES	DAILY DOSE	GENERAL INFO
MAGNESIUM			
Helps maintain normal muscle and nerve function, keeps heart rhythm steady, supports a healthy immune system, and keeps bones strong. Also helps regulate blood sugar levels, promotes normal blood pressure, and may manage disorders such as hypertension, cardiovascular disease and diabetes.	Fresh green veggies, spinach, beans, peas, nuts and seeds, and whole unrefined grains.	320 mg	Helps with absorption of calcium. Taking some medicines may result in magnesium deficiency: certain diuretics, antibiotics and medications taken to treat cancer.
PHOSPHORUS			
Critical for energy storage, metabolism, the utilization of many B-complex vitamins, proper muscle and nerve function, and for maintaining calcium balance.	Milk, cheese, dried beans, peas, colas, nuts, peanut butter.	700 mg	Potassium-sparing diuretics taken together with a phosphate may result in high blood levels of potassium.

BODY BENEFITS	FOOD SOURCES	DAILY DOSE	GENERAL INFO
POTASSIUM			
Necessary for the building of muscle, and for normal body growth. Assists in carbohydrate metabolism, and controls body water balance.	Apricots, bananas, all meats, soy products, broccoli, peas, lima beans, tomatoes, sweet potatoes, cantaloupe, kiwi, prunes, milk, yogurt.	4.7 mg	Diuretics, laxatives and steroids can cause loss of potassium.
SELENIUM			
Demonstrates antioxidant properties. Deficiency may affect thyroid function.	Liver, shellfish, salmon, tuna, halibut, alfalfa, radishes, onions, chives, brewer's yeast, wheat germ, butter, garlic, raisins, walnuts and sunflower seeds.	55 mg	Selenium levels may vary, and may be related to estrogen status.
ZINC			
May help keep the immune system functioning properly; necessary for the functioning of more than 300 different enzymes.	Legumes, meats, nuts, whole grains, oysters, sage, pumpkin seeds.	30 mg daily for 14 days for immune function	May cause nausea, vomiting or diarrhea.

BODY BENEFITS	FOOD SOURCES	DAILY DOSE	GENERAL INFO
OMEGA-3 FATTY ACIDS			
May assist in keeping triglyceride and cholesterol levels normal. Can reduce the risk of nonfatal heart attacks and help reduce inflammation. Recent trials report a small reduction in blood pressure.	Fish oil, walnuts, canola and soy oil, flax seeds, pumpkin seeds, fish (herring, salmon, bass, rainbow trout and sardines).	0.3–0.5 grams per day, or 2–3 servings of fish weekly	May exaggerate the effects of drugs that may also affect blood pressure. Can inhibit blood clotting. Consult with your doctor if you're taking omega-3 and you have a chronic blood disorder.
FLAXSEED			
Can be used as a laxative. There are unproven claims that associate flaxseed with improved cardiovascular outcomes.	Purchase at health food store.	10-250 grams daily	Contains soluble fiber; take with plenty of water. Do not take flaxseed at the same time as any conventional medication. It can lower the body's ability to absorb oral medications, and supplements. Take supplements 1-2 hours before taking flaxseed.

Sources: National Academy of Sciences, National Institutes of Health, and the RDA (recommended dietary allowances).

SOURCES

Institute of Medicine of the National Academies. *Dietary supplements: A framework for evaluating safety.* Washington, D.C: The National Academies; 2009. Available at: http://www.iom.edu/CMS/3788/4605/19578.aspx.

Sareen, S.S., J.L. Smith, et al. *Advanced nutrition and human metabolism, 5th ed.* Belmont, CA: Wadsworth, Cengage Learning; 2009.

National Institutes of Health. Dietary supplement use & safety. *Office of Dietary Supplements.* Available at: http://dietary-supplements.info.nih.gov.

U.S. Department of Agriculture, U.S. Department of Health and Human Services. *Nutrition and your health: Dietary guidelines for Americans 2005.* Washington, D.C: USDA Publication; 2005. Available at: http://www.health.gov/DietaryGuidelines

Non-Surgical Cosmetic Treatments

BRANDS	TARGET	PROCEDURE

ABLATIVE TREATMENTS
WORK BY DAMAGING THE SKIN'S SURFACE

LASER RESURFACING

Skin receives intense beams of light that travel in one direction. All tissue is treated. Skin layers are vaporized.

BRANDS	TARGET	PROCEDURE
CO2 Pulse Laser YAG Laser	Wrinkles around mouth and eyes, brown spots, sun damage, acne scarring, skin tone.	Laser hand piece moved over entire face 45 minutes up to $1\frac{1}{2}$ hours, local anesthesia is used in combination with oral sedatives.

LASER FRACTIONAL RESURFACING

Only a fraction of the skin receives the laser light.

BRANDS	TARGET	PROCEDURE
Fraxel Active FX	Wrinkles, acne scars, sun damage, brown spots, skin tightening, smoothing skin's texture.	Tiny microscopic wounds within the skin generate a wound-healing process that results in the coagulation of collagen fibers in the skin. Session lasts 10-30 minutes. Topical numbing cream is applied an hour prior.

RECOVERY	LONGEVITY	COST
	ABLATIVE TREATMENTS	

LASER RESURFACING

| Variable usually 10-21 days. Redness may last 2-3 months. | Long-lasting | $2,400-$5,000 |

LASER FRACTIONAL RESURFACING

| 3-5 days with 1 week of peeling, and some swelling and redness for up to 3 weeks after procedure. | Long-lasting. Additional treatments are recommended. Results do not equal the CO2 or YAG above. | $750-$1,100 per treatment |

BRANDS	TARGET	PROCEDURE

CHEMICAL PEELS

Induce exfoliation through application of various chemical agents.

BRANDS	TARGET	PROCEDURE
Glycolic, lactic or fruit acid (AHAs, alpha hydroxy acids) (Light peel)	Dull uneven skin, reduce effects of sun damage, improve acne scars, some types of brown imperfections and fine wrinkles.	Mild Alpha Hydroxyl Acid applied to entire face. No anesthesia needed. Lasts 30 minutes or more.
TCA peel (medium to deep peel) Trichloroacetic acid. Good for treating darker skin – sometimes called a Blue Peel.	Aggressive repair of sun-damaged skin, soften fine wrinkles, lessen brown discolorations, tighten skin, acne scars, large pores.	Peel applied directly to entire face. Can last 30 minutes up to 3 hours, depending on coverage.
Phenol Peel (deepest peel)	For deeper wrinkles from sun exposure or treat skin wrinkling around the lips and chin area.	1-2 hour procedure. There may be some discomfort, can be controlled with medication.

DERMABRASION

Uses a small, rapidly spinning wheel with a roughened surface – similar to fine-grade sandpaper – to abrade the skin, removing its upper layers.

BRANDS	TARGET	PROCEDURE
Rotary Abrasive Instrument	Acne scars, wrinkles, brown spots, sun damage.	High-speed rotary abrasive instrument used over entire face. Can last minutes to an hour.

RECOVERY	LONGEVITY	COST
		CHEMICAL PEELS
No downtime. May feel mild tingling during procedure.	May need multiple treatments.	$200-$900
2-3 days	May need multiple treatments.	$1,500-$2,500
1-2 weeks	Long-lasting.	$3,500-$5,000
		DERMABRASION
7-10 days	Long-lasting. Avoid sunlight for 3-6 months. May need multiple sessions.	$200+

BRANDS	TARGET	PROCEDURE

MICRO-DERMABRASION

Microscopic diamond chips smooth away superficial fine lines. Stimulates skin cells and collagen.

Micro-dermabrasion Facial	Minor fine lines, crow's feet, uneven skin, age spots and acne scars.	Hand piece emits crystals onto the surface of the skin, creating a polishing process. Lasts 30 minutes to an hour. No anesthetic required.

NON-ABLATIVE TREATMENTS
DO NOT DAMAGE THE TOP LAYER OF SKIN.

RADIO FREQUENCY

Uses a radio frequency instead of laser energy to heat the dermis while cooling and protecting the epidermis (top layer of skin).

Thermage (works on dark and light skin types)	Smooth wrinkles, tighten and lift skin.	Treatment tip heats and cools skin.
Polaris	Wrinkles, skin tightening	Radio frequency energy and light energy stimulate collagen production.
Aluma	Wrinkles, skin tightening	Hand piece moves over dermis of the skin, then suctions up the skin in the treatment, and the radio frequency waves are sent to the suctioned skin. No pain. Lasts 15-45 minutes.

RECOVERY	LONGEVITY	COST

MICRO-DERMABRASION

| No downtime. | Temporary results.

May need multiple sessions at 2-3 week intervals. | $150+ |

NON-ABLATIVE TREATMENTS

RADIO FREQUENCY

3-7 days of swelling. Redness may occur for a few hours after treatment.	Can last up to 5 years. Causes redness and swelling.	$1000-$5000 You may need more than one session.
None. Minor swelling after procedure.	4-5 treatments suggested, 3 weeks apart. Long-lasting.	$500-$5000
No downtime.	Six sessions are recommended, one per week.	$300 per treatment.

BRANDS	TARGET	PROCEDURE

INTENSE PULSED LIGHT (IPL)

Uses multiple wavelengths of light directed to the upper skin while delivering thermal energy to deeper layers. Reported to stimulate dermis for a collagen-producing effect.

BRANDS	TARGET	PROCEDURE
Photo Facial Foto Facial PhotoDerm Epilight	Brown spots, rosacea, broken capillaries, spider veins, redness, facial flushing and pigmentation.	Entire face, 30-45 minutes, patient feels snapping like a little rubber band.

LASER NON-ABLATIVE

BRANDS	TARGET	PROCEDURE
CoolTouch	Fine lines, brown spots, scarring, acne scars, skin tightening.	Uses a cooling spray before each pulse of infrared laser, protecting the top layer of skin. 15 minutes to 1 hour. Minimal discomfort.

DERMAL FILLERS

Product is injected into skin. Enhances soft tissue volume to smooth wrinkles or add fullness.

BRANDS	TARGET	PROCEDURE
Zyderm and Zyplast (collagen derived from purified bovine, cow, collagen)	Wrinkles around eyes, frown lines, scars and lip enhancement.	Injections under the area being treated. May feel some pain. Less than 1 hour.
Restylane and Hylaform (non-animal-based hyaluronic acid)	Treatment for mild-to-moderate facial creases, smile lines, and lips.	Injections under the area being treated. May feel some pain. Less than 1 hour.

RECOVERY	LONGEVITY	COST

INTENSE PULSED LIGHT (IPL)

| Redness may occur after treatment. No downtime. | Can last up to 5 years. Causes redness and swelling. | $1000-$5000 You may need more than one session. |

LASER NON-ABLATIVE

| No downtime. Redness may occur after treatment lasting a few hours. | 3 to 6 treatments over 2 to 4 weeks recommended. | $250-$500 per treatment. |

DERMAL FILLERS

| Redness and swelling at site may last a few hours after treatment. | Lasts 3-4 months (Potential for allergic reaction.) | $400-$500 per syringe. |
| Redness, bruising and swelling at injection site may last a few hours. | 4-6 months or more. | $550+ per syringe. |

BRANDS	TARGET	PROCEDURE
Radiesse Radiance (calcium hydroxylapatite)	Smile and frown lines, lines around eyes and lips.	Same. Less than 1 hour.
Self-donated fat injections	Restore facial fat loss. Used for lips, frown lines, and facial contouring.	Inject self-donated fat from abdomen, buttocks or thighs to area needing treatment. Lasts 30 minutes to 1 hour.

RELAXER

Restricts muscle action that results in facial creases. Botox is a protein derived from botulism toxin that is injected underneath the skin.

Botox	Softens wrinkles. Common on frown lines and crow's feet.	Injections under the skin at site of wrinkle, takes 30 minutes.

TOPICAL APPLICATION

Use topical products to smooth skin

Retinols Tretinoin	Smooth skin tone, and soften fine wrinkles.	Self-applied

HAIR REMOVAL - ELECTROLYSIS

Electrolysis unit	Hair removal	Fine electrode inserted into each hair follicle.

RECOVERY	LONGEVITY	COST
Bruising, swelling and redness at injection site may last for a few hours.	12 months and more, but may need touch-ups.	$800+ per treatment.
Swelling and bruising: Minor treatment 1-4 days; extensive 7-14 days.	May need follow-up treatments, since body can reabsorb its own tissue.	$400-$5,000

RELAXER

Slight numbness and bruising at injection site can last a few hours. 24-48 hours for sensitive patients.	3-6 months must repeat treatment.	$300-$500 per area

TOPICAL APPLICATION

None		$10-$80

HAIR REMOVAL - ELECTROLYSIS

None	3+ sessions required	$25-$150 per hour

BRANDS	TARGET	PROCEDURE

HAIR REMOVAL – LASER
Uses light pulse directed at hair follicle.

PhotoDerm HR	Hair removal	Light pulse directed at hair follicle. 1-2 hours.

SPIDER VEINS – SCLEROTHERAPY
Inject solution to collapse the vein

Sclerosing agent	Spider veins	Solution is injected into the veins, causing the vein to turn white then gradually disappear. Lasts 30 minutes to an hour. Minor discomfort.

SPIDER VEINS – LASER
Uses low-energy laser. The laser energy passes through the skin, being absorbed by the pigment in the hair follicle.

Laser	Spider veins	Lasts 30 minutes to an hour. No anesthesia needed in most cases. Minimal discomfort.

RECOVERY	LONGEVITY	COST

HAIR REMOVAL – LASER

| None | 3+ sessions required | $325+ |

SPIDER VEINS – SCLEROTHERAPY

| None | 3+ treatments to eliminate 60-90% of spider veins. | $200-$500 |

SPIDER VEINS – LASER

| None | Multiple sessions needed. Sometimes there is a temporary slight reddening of the treated area. | $400-$1,000 |

SOURCES

DiAmico, R.A., R. Saltz, et al. Plastic reconstruction surgery. *Plastic and Reconstructive Surgery.* 2008; 121(5): 1787–92.

The American Society for Aesthetic Plastic Surgery. Choose a procedure. Surgery.org. Available at: **http://www.surgery.org/public/procedures.**

APPENDIX D

Converting to Metric

VOLUME MEASUREMENT CONVERSIONS	
U.S.	**METRIC**
1/4 teaspoon	1.25 ml
1/2 teaspoon	2.5 ml
3/4 teaspoon	3.75 ml
1 teaspoon	5 ml
1 tablespoon	15 ml
1/4 cup	62.5 ml
1/2 cup	125 ml
3/4 cup	187.5 ml
1 cup	250 ml

WEIGHT CONVERSION MEASUREMENTS

U.S.	METRIC
1 ounce	28.4 g
8 ounces	227.5 g
16 ounces (1 pound)	455 g

COOKING TEMPERATURE CONVERSIONS

CELSIUS/CENTIGRADE	FAHRENHEIT
0°C and 100°C are arbitrarily placed at the melting and boiling points of water and standard to the metric system.	Fahrenheit established 0°F as the stabilized temperature when equal amounts of ice, water and salt are mixed.

To convert temperatures in Fahrenheit to Celsius, use this formula: $C = (F - 32) \times 0.5555$

So, for example, if you are baking at 350°F and want to know that temperature in Celsius, use this calculation:
$C = (350 - 32) \times 0.5555 = 176.66°C$

HELPFUL WEB SITES

The Menopause Makeover support, tips and information:
www.MenopauseMakeover.com

North American Menopause Society: www.menopause.org

The International Menopause Society: www.imsociety.org

Summary of Hormone Therapy Findings from the International
Menopause Society:
www.imsociety.org/pdf_files/comments_and_press_statements/ims_
press_statement_13_05_08.pdf

The Society for Women's Health Research:
www.womenshealthresearch.org

Osteoporosis and Related Bone Disease National Resource Center:
www.osteo.org

Calculate your osteoporosis risk: www.shef.ac.uk/FRAX

National Osteoporosis Foundation: www.nof.org

National Center for Complementary and Alternative Medicine:
nccam.nih.gov

Complementary and Alternative Medicine (CAM) for health-care
professionals and the public: camline.ca

American College of Obstetricians and Gynecologists (ACOG):
www.acog.org

National Institute on Aging, NIA Information Center:
www.nih.gov/nia

Women's Health Initiative: www.nhlbi.nih.gov/whi

The American Society for Aesthetic Plastic Surgery:
www.surgery.org

Menopause Humor and Information: www.minniepauz.com

Easy, low-calorie recipes: www.hungry-girl.com

Calorie food information: www.calorie-count.com

Menopause Entertainment: www.menopausethemusical.com

National Association of Baby Boomer Women:
www.nabbw.com

Medication, supplements and cosmetics safety information:
www.fda.gov/medwatch/SAFETY.htm

National Health Products Directorate (NHPD):
www.hc-sc.gc.ca/index_eng.php

Health Information: medlineplus.gov

Cosmetic safety database: www.cosmeticdatabase.com

Nutritional Scoring System: www.nuval.com

REFERENCES

CHAPTER 1

Speroff, L. and F.A. Fritz. *Clinical gynecologic endocrinology and infertility.* Philadelphia, PA: Lippincott Williams & Wilkins; 2004.

The North American Menopause Society. Menopause practice: *A clinician's Guide, 3rd ed.* Cleveland, OH: The North American Menopause Society; 2007.

Santoro, N. Symptoms of menopause: hot flashes. *Clinical Obstetrics Gynecology.* 2008; 51(3): 539–48.

Harrison, S. and W. Bergfeld. Diffuse hair loss: its triggers and management. *Cleveland Clinic Journal of Medicine.* 2009; 76(6): 361–7.

Somani, N., S. Harrison and W.F. Bergfeld. The clinical evaluation of hirsutism. *Dermatologic Therapy.* 2008; 21(5): 376–91.

Davis, M. and R. Kroll. Testosterone Improves Sexual Function in Women Not Taking Estrogen. The North American Menopause Society, *First to Know.* December 23, 2008; 359: 2005–2017.

CHAPTER 2

Sturdee, D.W. *The facts of hormone therapy for menopausal women.* New York: The Parthenon Publishing Group; 2004.

International Menopause Society. Recommendations on postmenopausal therapy. *Climacteric.* 2007; 10: 181–94. Available at: http://www.imsociety.org/ pdf_files/ims_recommendations/ims_updated_recommendations_on_postmenopausal_hormone_therapy_27_02_07.pdf

The North American Menopause Society. *Early menopause guidebook, 6 ed.* Cleveland, OH: The North American Menopause Society; 2007.

National Institute on Aging. What can you do for hot flashes and other menopausal symptoms. Available at: http://www.nia.nih.gov/Healthinformation/Publications/Menopause/what.htm.htm

Suckling, J., A. Lethaby and R. Kennedy. Local estrogen for vaginal atrophy in postmenopausal women. Cochrane Database of Systematic Reviews. 2006; (4): CD001500.

Hemelaar, M., M. van der Mooren, et al. Effects of transdermal and oral postmenopausal hormone therapy on vascular function: A randomized, placebo-controlled study in healthy postmenopausal women. *Menopause*. 2005; 12(5): 526–35.

Rinaldi, M., A. Cagnacci, et al. Neutral effect of prolonged transdermal hormone therapy on liver function of postmenopausal women with chronic active hepatitis. *Menopause*. 2005; 12(5): 619–22.

Wingert, P. and B. Kantrowitz. Are bioidentical hormones safe? *Newsweek*. February 7, 2008.

Simon, J.A. *Understanding the controversy: Hormone testing and bioidentical hormones*. 17th Annual Meeting of the North American Menopause Society; 2006.

Lui, L., Y.S. Dong, et al. Biotransformation of steroidal saponins in *Dioscorea zingiberensis* C.H. Wright to diosgenin by *Trichoderma harzianum*. *Applied Microbiology Biotechnology*. July 2009. [Epub ahead of print] PMID: 19578845

The North American Menopause Society. *Menopause practice: A clinician's guide, 3rd ed.* Cleveland, OH: The North American Menopause Society; 2007.

Vogel, J., *Understanding the controversy: Hormone testing and bioidentical hormones: Selecting bioidentical hormone therapy.* 17th Annual Meeting of the North American Menopause Society; 2006.

U.S. Food and Drug Administration. *Limited FDA survey of compounded drug products.* June 18, 2009. Available at: http://www.fda.gov/Drugs/GuidanceComplianceRegulatoryInformation/PharmacyCompounding/ucm155725.htm

Richardson, M.K. *Understanding the controversy: Hormone testing and bioidentical hormones: Counseling patients about bioidentical hormone therapy.* 17th Annual Meeting of the North American Menopause Society; 2006.

Allen, Loyd V. *Understanding the controversy: Hormone testing and bioidentical hormones: Compounding practices and controversies.* 17th Annual Meeting of the North American Menopause Society; 2006.

The Endocrine Society. *Bioidentical hormones position statement.* October 2006. Available at: http://www.endo-society.org/advocacy/policy/upload/BH_Position_Statement_final_10_25_06_w_Header.pdf

Patsner, B., *Understanding the controversy: Hormone testing and bioidentical hormones: Regulatory issues of compounding drugs.* 17th Annual Meeting of the North American Menopause Society; 2006.

Rinaldi, M., A. Cagnacci, et al. Neutral effect of prolonged transdermal hormone therapy on liver function of postmenopausal women with chronic active hepatitis. *Menopause.* 2005; 12(5): 619–22.

Bachmann, G. and R.A. Lobo, et al. Efficacy of low-dose estradiol vaginal tablets in the treatment of atrophic vaginitis: A randomized controlled trial. *Obstetrics and Gynecology.* 2008; 111(1): 67–76.

Cirigliano, M., Bioidentical hormone therapy: a review of the evidence. *Journal of Women's Health.* 2007; 16(5): 500–31.

Sites, C.K., Bioidentical hormones for menopausal therapy. *Women's Health (Lond, Engl).* 2008; 4(2): 163–71.

Rodgers, A.K. and T. Falcone. Treatment strategies for endometriosis. *Expert Opinion on Pharmacotherapy.* 2008; 9(2): 243–55.

Wingert, P. and B. Kantrowitz. *Is it hot in here? Or is it me? The complete guide to menopause.* New York: Workman Publishing Company, Incorporated; 2006.

Department of Health and Human Services, National Institutes of Health, National Heart, Lung and Blood Institute. *Questions and answers about the WHI postmenopausal hormone therapy trials.* April 2004. Available at: http://www.nhlbi.nih.gov/whi/whi_faq.htm

Haimov-Kochman, R. and D. Hochner-Celnikier. *Are there second thoughts about the results of the WHI study?* Acta Obstetricia et Gynecologica Scandinavica. 2006;85(4): 387–393.

Pines, A., D.W. Sturdee, et al. More data on hormone therapy and coronary heart disease: Comments on recent publications for the WHI and nurses' health study. *Climacteric.* 2006; 9(2): 75–6.

Pines, A., D.W. Sturdee, et al. HRT in the early menopause: Scientific evidence and common perceptions. *Climacteric.* 2008; 11(4): 267–72.

Pines, A., D.W. Sturdee, et al. The heart of the WHI study: Time for hormone therapy policies to be revised. *Climacteric.* 2007; 10: 267–269.

Palacios, S. Advances in hormone replacement therapy: Making menopause manageable. *BMC Women's Health.* 2008; 8:22.

Furness, S., H. Roberts, et al. Hormone therapy in postmenopausal women and risk of endometrial hyperplasia. *Cochrane Database Systematic Reviews.* 2009; (2): CD000402.

Mascitelli, L., M.R. Goldstein, et al. Questioning the cardioprotective action of hormone replacement therapy in postmenopausal women. *Journal of Cardiovascular Medicine* (Hagerstown). 2009; 10(8): 657–8.

Pines, A. and D. Sturdee, et al. WHI and breast cancer. *Climacteric*. April 11, 2006.

Seidlova-Wuttke, D. and O. Hesse, et al. Evidence for selective estrogen receptor modular activity in a black cohosh (Cimicifuga racemosa) extract: Comparison with estradiol-17beta. *European Journal of Endocrinology*. 2003; 149(4): 351–62.

The North American Menopause Society. Do mother nature's treatments help hot flashes? *Menopause Flashes*. 2008; 3(1): 7.

DeKosky, S.T., J.D. Williamson, et al. Gingko biloba does not prevent dementia. *JAMA: the journal of the American Medical Association*. 2008; 300: 2253–2262.

Natural Standard Research Collaboration. Ginseng (American Ginseng, Asian Ginseng, Chinese Ginseng, Korean Red Ginseng, *Panax ginseng*, Panax spp. Including *P. Ginseng* C.C. Meyer and *P. quinquefolius L.*, excluding *Eleutherococcus senticosus*). March 1, 2008. Available at: http://www.nlm.nih.gov/medlineplus/druginfo/natural/patient-ginseng.html

CHAPTER 3

Sternfeld, B., H. Wang, et al. Physical activity and changes in weight and waist circumference in midlife women: findings from the study of women's health across the nation. *American Journal of Epidemiology*. 2004; 160(9): 912–22.

Liu, Y., and J. Ding, et al. Relative androgen excess and increased cardiovascular risk after menopause: A hypothesized relation. *American Journal of Epidemiology*. 2001; 154(6): 489–94.

Gropper, S.S., J.L. Smith, et al. *Advanced nutrition and human metabolism, 5th ed.* Belmont, CA: Wadsworth, Cengage Learning; 2009.

U.S. Food and Drug Administration. Talking about trans fat: What you need to know. May 2006. Available at: http://www.fda.gov/Food/ResourcesForYou/Consumers/ucm079609.htm

Schryver, T. and C. Smith. Participants' willingness to consume soy foods for lowering cholesterol and receive counseling on cardiovascular disease by nutrition professionals. *Public Health Nutrition*. 2006; 9(7): 866–74.

Nieves, J.W. Nutritional therapies (including fosteum). *Current Osteoporosis Reports*. 2009; 7(1): 5–11.

Zhang, X., X.O. Shu, et al. Prospective cohort study of soy food consumption and risk of bone fracture among postmenopausal women. *Archives of Internal Medicine*. 2005; 165(16): 1890–5.

Busko, M., and H. Nghlem. Diets with high omega-6:omega-3 ratios enhance risk for depression, inflammatory disease. *MedscapeCME*. April 26, 2007. Available at: http://cme.medscape.com/viewarticle/555736

Harris, W., and D. Mozaffarian, et al. Omega-6 fatty acids and risk for cardiovascular disease. *Circulation*. 2009; 119: 902–907.

American Heart Association. *Know your fats*. Available at: http://www.americanheart.org/presenter.jhtml?identifier=532

Kurtzweil, P. Help in preventing heart disease. U.S. Food and Drug Administration, *FDA Consumer*. December 1994. Available at: http://www.fda.gov.fdac.foodlabel/ heart.html

Kiecolt-Glaser, J.K., M.A. Belury, et al. Depressive symptoms, omega-6:omega-3 acids, and inflammation in older adults. *Psychosomatic Medicine*. 2007; 69(3): 217–24.

Mayo Clinic. Water: How much should you drink every day? *Mayoclinic.com*. Available at: http://www.mayoclinic.com/print/water/ NU00283/METHOD=print

National Institutes of Health. Drinking water. *Medline Plus*. July 6, 2009. Available at: http://www.nlm.nih.gov/medlineplus/drinkingwater.html

American Heart Association. *Tobacco industry's targeting of youth, minorities and women*. May 20, 2009. Available at: http://www.americanheart.org/presenter.jhtml?identifier=11226

Delichatsios, H.K. and F.K. Welty. Influence of the DASH diet and other low-fat, high-carbohydrate diets on blood pressure. *Current Atherosclerosis Reports*. 2005; 7(6): 446–54.

Jacobson, M. Salt: The Forgotten Killer. *Center for Science in the Public Interest*. December 2008. Available at: http://cspinet.org/new/pdf/ saltupdatedec08.pdf

Mayo Clinic. Sodium: Are you getting too much? *MayoClinic.com*. May 23, 2008. Available at: http://www.mayoclinic.com/health/sodium/NU00284

U.S. Department of Health and Human Services. Your guide to lowering your blood pressure with DASH. *National Institutes of Health*. April 2006. Available at: http://www.nhlbi.nih.gov/health/public/heart/hbp/dash/ new_dash.pdf

Lichtenstein, A.H., H. Rasmussen, et al. Modified MyPyramid for older adults. *The Journal of Nutrition*. 2008; 138: 5–11.

U.S. Department of Agriculture. Search the USDA National Nutrient Database for standard reference. Nutrient lists. Nutrient Data Laboratory. Available at: http://www.nal.usda.gov/fnic/foodcomp/search

U.S. Department of Agriculture. MyPyramid.gov: Steps to a healthier you. MyPyramid.gov. *United States Department of Agriculture.* June 26, 2009. Available at: http://www.mypyramid.gov

The North American Menopause Society. *Menopause practice: A clinician's guide, 3rd ed.* Cleveland, OH: The North American Menopause Society; 2007.

CHAPTER 4

U.S. Department of Health and Human Services. Physical activity has many health benefits. *Physical activity guidelines for Americans.* October 16, 2008. Available at: http://www.health.gov./PAGuidleines/guidelines/chapter2.aspx

The North American Menopause Society. Menopause practice: *A clinician's guide, 3rd ed.* Cleveland, OH: The North American Menopause Society; 2007.

Lloyd-Jones, D., R. Adams, et al. Heart disease and stroke statistics—2008 update. *Circulation.* 2009; 119(3): 480–6.

U.S. Department of Health and Human Services. The heart truth for women: An action plan. *The heart truth.* Available at: http://www.hhs.state.ne.us/hew/owh/docs/ActionPlan.pdf

Ness, J., W.S. Aronow, et al. Use of hormone replacement therapy by postmenopausal women after publication of the Women's Health Initiative trial. *The Journals of Gerontology. Series A, Biological Sciences and Medical Sciences.* 2005; 60(4): 460–2.

Mesch, V.R., N.O. Siseles, et al. Androgens in relationship to cardio-vascular risk factors in the menopausal transition. *Climacteric.* 2008; 11(6): 509–17.

Gaddam, K.K., A. Verma, et al. Hypertension and cardiac failure in its various forms. *The Medical Clinics of North America.* 2009; 93(3): 665–80.

Lee, L.V. and J.M. Foody. Cardiovascular disease in women. *Current Atherosclerosis Reports.* 2008; 10(4): 295–302.

U.S. Department of Health and Human Services. What is high blood pressure? *National Heart, Lung and Blood Institute, Disease and Conditions Index.* Available at: http://www.nhlbi.nih.gov/health/dci/Diseases/Hbp/HBP_WhatIs.html

National Institutes of Health. Your guide to lowering high blood pressure. What is blood pressure? *National Heart, Lung and Blood Institute.* Available at: http://www.nhlbi.nih.gov/hbp/bp/bp.htm

National Institutes of Health, Department of Health and Human Services. Osteoporosis: Peak bone mass in women. *National Institute of Arthritis and Musculoskeletal and Skin Diseases.* May 2009. Available at: http://www.niams.nih.gov/Health_Info/Bone/Osteoporosis/bone_mass.asp

U.S. Department of Health and Human Services. Your guide to physical activity and your heart. *National Heart, Lung and Blood Institute.* January 2008. Available at: http://www.nhlbi.nih.gov/health/public/heart/obesity/phy_active.pdf

Poehlman, E.T., W.F. Denino, et al. Effects of endurance and resistance training on total daily energy expenditure in young women: A controlled randomized trial. *The Journal of Clinical Endocrinology and Metabolism.* 2002; 87(3): 1004–9.

Wang, Z., S. Heshka, et al. Resting energy expenditure: Systematic organization and critique of prediction methods. *Obesity Research.* 2001; 9(5): 331–6.

U.S. Department of Health and Human Services. *Dietary guidelines for Americans, 2005.* Washington, DC: U.S. Government Printing Office; 2005.

National Institute on Aging. *Exercise and physical activity: Your everyday guide from the National Institute on aging.* Bethesda, MD: 2008.

Iwao, S., N. Iwao, et al. Does waist circumference add to the predictive power of the body mass index for coronary risk? *Obesity Research.* 2001; 9(11): 685–695.

Dennison, Haines C. Losing weight. National Institutes of Health. *Medline Plus.* 2007. Available at: http://www.nlm.nih.gov/medlineplus/ency/article/001940.htm

Del Corral, Pedro, P. Chandler-Laney, et al. Effect of dietary adherence with or without exercise on weight loss: A mechanistic approach to a global problem. *Journal of Clinical Endocrinology & Metabolism.* 2009; 94(5): 1602–1607.

Department of Health and Family Services, State of Wisconsin. Calories burned per hour. 2005. *Department of Health and Family Services.* Available at: http://dhs.wisconsin.gov/health/physicalactivity/pdf_files/Caloriesperhour.pdf

Topol, E., M.D. Eisner, et al. *Cleveland Clinic heart book: The definitive guide for the entire family from the nation's leading heart center.* New York: Hyperion; 2000.

Gersch, B.J. Mayo *Clinic heart book, revised edition: The ultimate guide to heart health.* New York: William Morrow. 2000.

American Heart Association. One-mile fitness calculator. *Learn and live*. 2008. Available at: http://www.americanheart.org/presenter.jhtml?identifier=3046243

CHAPTER 5

The North American Menopause Society. *Menopause Practice: A Clinician's Guide, 3rd ed.* Cleveland, OH: The North American Menopause Society; 2007.

American Society for Aesthetic Plastic Surgery. Cosmetic plastic surgery research statistics and trends for 2001–2007. *Plastic Surgery Research.info.* February 25, 2008. Available at: http://www.cosmeticplasticsurgerystatistics.com/statistics.html

U.S. Census Bureau. Industry statistics sampler: NAICS 315231 women's and girls' cut and sew lingerie, loungewear, and nightwear manufacturing. *Economic census 2002.* 2004. Available at: http://www.census.gov/epcd/ec97/industry/E315231.htm

The bra guide. Are you wearing the right bra size? bra calculator. *Your source for bra info.* Available at: http://bra.and.bras.googlepages.com/bra_size_calculator.html

CHAPTER 6

The North American Menopause Society. *Menopause practice: A clinician's guide, 3rd ed.* Cleveland, OH: The North American Menopause Society; 2007.

Brizendine, L. *The Female Brain.* New York: Broadway Books; 2006.

National Institute of Mental Health. Depression: A treatable illness (fact sheet). Reprinted 2004. *Transforming the understanding and treatment of mental illness through research.* Available at: http://www.nimh.nih.gov/health/publications/ depression-a-treatable-illness-fact-sheet/index.shtml

Speroff, L. and F.A. Fritz. Clinical gynecologic endocrinology and infertility. Philadelphia, PA: Lippincott Williams & Wilkins; 2004.

CHAPTER 7

Brizendine, L. *The Female Brain.* New York: Broadway Books; 2006.

The North American Menopause Society. *Menopause practice: A clinician's guide, 3rd ed.* Cleveland, OH: The North American Menopause Society; 2007.

Amato, P. Categories of female sexual dysfunction. *Obstetrics and Gynecology Clinics of North America.* 2006; 33(4): 527–34.

Tessler, Lindau S., P. Schumm, et al. A study of sexuality and health among older adults in the United States. *The New England Journal of Medicine.* 2007; 357(8): 762–774.

Wingert, P. and B. Kantrowitz. *Is it hot in here? Or is it me? The complete guide to menopause.* New York: Workman Publishing Company, Incorporated; 2006.

Shifren, J.L., G.D. Braunstein, et al. Transdermal testosterone treatment in women with impaired sexual function after oophorectomy. *The New England Journal of Medicine.* 2000; 343(10): 682–8.

CHAPTER 8

Daley, A.J., H.J. Stokes-Lampard, et al. Exercise to reduce vasomotor and other menopausal symptoms: A review. *Maturitas.* 2009; 63(3): 176–80.

Chiesa, A. Zen meditation: An integration of current evidence. *Journal of Alternative and Complementary Medicine.* 2009; 15(5): 585–92.

King, M.S., T. Carr, et al. Transcendental meditation, hypertension and heart disease. *Australian Family Physician.* 2002; 31(2): 164–8.

Lutz, A., L.L. Greischar, et al. Long-term meditators self-induce high-amplitude gamma synchrony during mental practice. *Proceeding of the National Academy of Sciences of the United States of America.* 2004; 101(46): 16369–79.

Davidson, R.J., J. Kabat-Zinn, et al. Alterations in brain and immune function produced by mindfulness meditation. *Psychosomatic Medicine.* 2003; 65(4): 564–70.

CHAPTER 9

Dictionary.com. Happiness. *Dictionary.com.* Available at: http://dictionary.reference.com/browse/happiness

CHAPTER 10

Bray G.A. and D.S. Gray. Obesity. Part II—Treatment. *The Western Journal of Medicine.* 1988; 149(5): 555–71.

National Heart Lung and Blood Institute. Classification of overweight and obesity by BMI, waist circumference, and associated disease risks. *Obesity Education Initiative.* Available at: http://www.nhlbi.nih.gov/health/public/heart/obesity/ lose_wt/bmi_dis.htm

Ehrman, J.K., P.M. Gordon, et al. *Clinical exercise physiology.* Champaign, IL: Human Kinetics; 2009.

Gropper, S.S., J.L. Smith, et al. *Advanced nutrition and human metabolism*. Belmont, CA: Wadsworth Cengage Learning; 2009.

Snow, V., P. Barry, et al. Pharmacologic and surgical management of obesity in primary care: A clinical care practice from the American College of Physicians. *Annals of Internal Medicine*. 2005; 142(7): 525–531.

American College of Physicians. Overweight/obesity and weight control. Available at: http://www.acponline.org/patients_families/diseases_conditions/obesity

American College of Physicians. 100 million adult Americans are overweight and at risk of serious disease. *Internal medicine doctor for adults*. Available at: http://www.acponline.org/patients_families/pdfs/health/obesity.pdf

National Institutes of Health. Obesity, physical activity, and weight-control glossary. *An information service of the National Institute of Diabetes and Digestive and Kidney Diseases (NIDDK)*. Available at: http://win.niddk.nih.gov/publications/glossary.htm

Boschmann, M., J. Steiniger, et al. Water-induced thermogenesis. *The Journal of Clinical Endocrinology and Metabolism*. 2003; 88(12): 6015–9.

Halton, T.L. and F.B. HU. The effects of high protein diets on thermogenesis, satiety and weight loss: A critical review. *Journal of the American College of Nutrition*. 2004; 23(5): 373–85.

CHAPTER 11

Ehrman, J.K., P.M. Gordon, et al. *Clinical exercise physiology*. Champaign, IL: Human Kinetics; 2009.

Gropper, S.S., J.L. Smith, et al. *Advanced nutrition and human metabolism*. Belmont, CA: Wadsworth Cengage Learning; 2009.

Body mass index chart. Partnership for healthy weight management. *Consumer.gov*. Available at: http://www.consumer.gov/weightloss/bmi.htm

U.S. Department of Health and Human Services. Facts about healthy weight. *National Heart, Lung and Blood Institute*. 2006. Available at: http://www.nhlbi.nih.gov/health/prof/heart/obesity/aim_kit/healthy_wt_facts.htm

U.S. Department of Health and Human Services. Weight and waist measurement: Tools for adults. *The Weight-control Information Network*. 2008. Available at: http://win.niddk.nih.gov/publications/tools.htm

Stob, N.R., C. Bell, et al. Thermic effect of food and beta-adrenergic thermogenic responsiveness in habitually exercising and sedentary healthy adult humans. *Journal of Applied Physiology*. 2007; 103(2): 616–22.

Tsai, A.G. and T.A. Wadden. Systematic review: An evaluation of major commercial weight loss programs in the United States. *Annals of Internal Medicine.* 2005; 142(1): 56–66.

Haskell, W.L., I.M. Lee, et al. Physical activity and public health: Updated recommendation for adults from the American College of Sports Medicine and the American Heart Association. *Medicine and Science in Sports Exercise.* 2007; 39(8): 1423–34.

Harris, A.J. and F.G. Benedict. A biometric study of human basal metabolism. *Proceedings of the National Academy of Sciences of the United States of America.* 1918; 4(12): 370–373.

CHAPTER 13

The North American Menopause Society. *Menopause practice: A clinician's guide, 3rd ed.* Cleveland, OH: The North American Menopause Society; 2007.

CHAPTER 14

Kuo, M.L., T.S. Huang, et al. Curcumin, an antioxidant and anti-tumor promoter, induces apoptosis in human leukemia cells. *Biochimica et Biophysica Acta.* 1996; 1317(2): 95–100.

Motterlini, R., R. Foresti, et al. Curcumin, an antioxidant and anti-inflammatory agent, induces heme oxygenase-1 and protects endothelial cells against oxidative stress. *Free Radical Biology & Medicine.* 2000; 28(8): 1303–12.

Mahmmoud, Y.A. Capsaicin stimulates uncoupled ATP hydrolysis by the sarcoplasmic reticulum calcium pump. *The Journal of Biological Chemistry.* 2008; 283(3): 21418–26.

Weisburger, J.H. Eat to live, not live to eat. *Nutrition.* 2000; 16(9): 767–73.

McShea, A., E. Ramiro-Puig, et al. Clinical benefit and preservation of flavonols in dark chocolate manufacturing. *Nutrition Reviews.* 2008; 66(11): 630–41.

Stibich, Mark. Health Benefits of Chocolate. *Longevity.* January 24, 2009. Available at: http://longevity.about.com/od/lifelongnutrition/p/chocolate.htm

Penumathsa, S.V. and N. Maulik. Resveratrol: A promising agent in promoting cardioprotection against coronary heart disease. *Canadian Journal of Physiology and Pharmacology.* 2009; 87(4): 275–86.

Calderon, A.I., B.J. Wright, et al. Screening antioxidants using LC-MS: Case study with cocoa. *The Journal of Agricultural and Food Chemistry.* 2009; 57(13): 5693–9.

Corti, R., A.J. Flammer, et al. Cocoa and cardiovascular health. *Circulation*. 2009; 119(10): 1433–41.

CHAPTER 15

Shen, W. and V. Stearns. Treatment strategies for hot flashes. *Expert Opinion on Pharmacotherapy*. 2009; 10(7): 1133–44.

APPENDIX

APPENDIX A

The North American Menopause Society. *Menopause practice: A clinician's guide, 3rd ed.* Cleveland, OH: The North American Menopause Society, 2009. Available at: http://www.menopause.org/htcharts.pdf

APPENDIX B

Institute of Medicine of the National Academies. *Dietary supplements: A framework for evaluating safety.* Washington, D.C: The National Academies; 2009. Available at: http://www.iom.edu/CMS/3788/4605/19578.aspx

Sareen, S.S., J.L. Smith, et al. *Advanced nutrition and human metabolism, 5th ed.* Belmont, CA: Wadsworth, Cengage Learning; 2009.

National Institutes of Health. Dietary supplement use & safety. *Office of Dietary Supplements.* Available at: http://dietary-supplements.info.nih.gov

U.S. Department of Agriculture, U.S. Department of Health and Human Services. Nutrition and your health: *Dietary guidelines for Americans 2005.* Washington, D.C: USDA Publication; 2005. Available at: http://www.health.gov/DietaryGuidelines

APPENDIX C

DiAmico, R.A., R. Saltz, et al. Plastic reconstruction surgery. Plastic and Reconstructive Surgery. 2008; 121(5): 1787–92.

The American Society for Aesthetic Plastic Surgery. Choose a procedure. *Surgery.org.* Available at: http://www.surgery.org/public/procedures

INDEX

ACKNOWLEDGMENTS

The Menopause Makeover had a five-year gestation period from its creation to becoming a book. This journey would not have been possible without the incredible support of my husband, Michael Becker. He worked tirelessly so I had the freedom to create, research and write this book, all the while loving me during moments of serious crankiness while going through one of the biggest changes in my life.

I would like to thank my mom and dad, Joyce and Stan Jonekos, for teaching me as a child that I could do anything. I never heard, "Girls don't do that." I always heard, "Go for it!" My brother, Stan Jonekos, always loved me, even when I got him in trouble.

This book would not be in your hands without Rick Broadhead, literary agent extraordinaire. I am forever grateful for Rick's incredible support, wisdom and belief in this book, and for securing the perfect publisher.

An enormous thank you to Deb Brody, executive editor at Harlequin, who had the vision to see that menopausal women needed a makeover action planner on their bookshelves, and invited *The Menopause Makeover* into the Harlequin nonfiction family. Sarah Pelz, editor at Harlequin, whose editorial advice honored the tone of this book, and who was fun to work with—thank you.

A big thank-you to Dr. Wendy Klein for the medical accuracy of this book. Dr. Klein is truly an advocate for women's health, as well as a woman of excellence, both personally and professionally.

Speaking of doctors, I must thank my own lifetime doctor, Dr. Josephine Hall. She has been a crusader for my health since I was 20 years old. Had it not been for my own absence from her care, I would not have had the menopause challenges I experienced.

A special thank-you to my good friends, Kathryn Hewitt, Terri Seifried and Sara Martin, who listened to me chatter on and on about menopause and offered their expertise when needed, usually at the last minute. And to my other close gal pals (Colleen, Sheri, Theresa, Sonya, Joan, Nancy, Pamela, Renay and Claire) going through menopause without a girlfriend is like getting married without a groom—it is just not possible.

I also thank Bethany Berndt-Shackelford who gave *The Menopause Makeover* book proposal a beautiful face with her incredible artwork. Thank you to Lisa Wallender, Judy Morton and Elyssia Stratton for doing the Menopause Makeover with great success and inspiring others by sharing their stories.

I would also like to thank Carol Peper, an incredible writer herself, for giving me support and encouragement from the beginning.

And finally, I would like to thank all the women I encountered on my journey who believed in *The Menopause Makeover*.

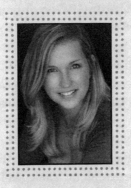

Staness Jonekos is an advocate for women's health, wellness and empowerment. Despite having a name that's derived from the man's name, Stanley, Staness has been a lifelong crusader for women. An award-winning television writer, producer and director, she was one of the original executive producers who launched the television network Oxygen Media, cofounded by Oprah Winfrey. Staness delivered five series and cocreated Oxygen Media's "Be Fearless" campaign to empower women.

Following her commitment for women's health, Staness coexecutive produced the premiere season of VH1's *Celebrity Fit Club,* and postproduced Lifetime's *Speaking of Women's Health.* She earned a Cindy Award for her role producing and directing an antismoking PSA for the State of California.

Prior credits include producer, director and/or writer for MTV's *Road Rules* (season 4, episode #407 won a Prism Award); ABC's half-hour reality pilot *Young Cops* and *Wallet Roulette,* WE's *Savvy,* A&E's *L.A. Detectives, Sons of Hollywood* and two-hour special *Conspiracies;* Discovery Channel's *IMPACT* and *Head to Head,* and Travel Channel's *Travel Daily.*

Staness Jonekos is president and founder of Krystal Productions, an award-winning film and video production company based in Los Angeles. Created in 1988, Krystal Productions provides film and video services for television programming, independent documentaries and commercials.

Staness holds a bachelor's degree in theater from UCLA and is an active member of the Producers Guild of America, the Academy of Television Arts & Sciences, the International Documentary Association, the North American Menopause Society and the International Menopause Society.

Currently writing her next nonfiction book and first novel, Staness lives in Los Angeles with her husband and German shepherd pup.